SELF-HEALING
WITH
REIKI

Penelope Quest is a Usui Reiki Master who has been practicing
Reiki since 1991 and teaching it since 1994. As a member of the
UK Reiki Federation, in 2005 she helped devise a core curriculum
for Reiki Practitioner training. Her bestselling Reiki titles,
Reiki for Life, The Basics of Reiki, Living the Reiki Way and
The Reiki Manual, have received international acclaim.

SELF-HEALING WITH REIKI

How to Create Wholeness,
Harmony & Balance
for Body, Mind & Spirit

PENELOPE QUEST

JEREMY P. TARCHER/PENGUIN
a member of Penguin Group (USA) Inc.
New York

JEREMY P. TARCHER/PENGUIN
Published by the Penguin Group
Penguin Group (USA) Inc., 375 Hudson Street, New York, New York 10014, USA •
Penguin Group (Canada), 90 Eglinton Avenue East, Suite 700, Toronto,
Ontario M4P 2Y3, Canada (a division of Pearson Penguin Canada Inc.) • Penguin Books Ltd,
80 Strand, London WC2R 0RL, England • Penguin Ireland, 25 St Stephen's Green,
Dublin 2, Ireland (a division of Penguin Books Ltd) • Penguin Group (Australia),
250 Camberwell Road, Camberwell, Victoria 3124, Australia (a division
of Pearson Australia Group Pty Ltd) • Penguin Books India Pvt Ltd, 11 Community Centre,
Panchsheel Park, New Delhi–110 017, India • Penguin Group (NZ),
67 Apollo Drive, Rosedale, North Shore 0632, New Zealand (a division of
Pearson New Zealand Ltd) • Penguin Books (South Africa) (Pty) Ltd, 24 Sturdee Avenue,
Rosebank, Johannesburg 2196, South Africa

Penguin Books Ltd, Registered Offices: 80 Strand, London WC2R 0RL, England

First published in Great Britain in 2003 by Judy Piatkus (Publishers) Limited.
First trade paperback edition published in 2009 by Piatkus.
First American edition published in 2012 by Tarcher/Penguin.
Copyright © 2003 by Penelope Quest

Most Tarcher/Penguin books are available at special quantity discounts for
bulk purchase for sales promotions, premiums, fund-raising, and educational
needs. Special books or book excerpts also can be created to fit specific needs.
For details, write Penguin Group (USA) Inc. Special Markets,
375 Hudson Street, New York, NY 10014.

Library of Congress Cataloging-in-Publication Data

Quest, Penelope.
Self-healing with reiki : how to create wholeness, harmony & balance for body, mind & spirit / Penelope
Quest.—1st American ed.
p.   cm.
Originally published: Great Britain : Judy Piatkus (Publishers) Limited, 2003.
ISBN 978-1-58542-905-9
1. Reiki (Healing system)   2. Self-care, Health.   I. Title.
RZ403.R45Q84   2012   2012012909
615.8'52—dc23

Printed in the United States of America
1 3 5 7 9 10 8 6 4 2

Book design by Briony Chappell
Illustrations by Rodney Paull

While the author has made every effort to provide accurate telephone numbers and Internet addresses at the time of publication, neither the publisher nor the author assumes any responsibility for errors, or for changes that occur after publication. Further, the publisher does not have any control over and does not assume any responsibility for author or third-party websites or their content.

Neither the publisher nor the author is engaged in rendering professional advice or services to the individual reader. The ideas, procedures, and suggestions contained in this book are not intended as a substitute for consulting with your physician. All matters regarding your health require medical supervision. Neither the author nor the publisher shall be liable or responsible for any loss or damage allegedly arising from any information or suggestion in this book.

CONTENTS

Disclaimer

This book gives nonspecific, general information to help you in your quest for physical fitness, good health and general well-being. It should not be relied on as a substitute for proper medical consultation. While all suggested treatments and techniques are offered in good faith, the author and publisher cannot accept responsibility for the results of your actions in using any of the information in this book for yourself, or for any illness arising out of the failure to seek medical advice from a doctor.

ACKNOWLEDGMENTS

I would like to express my heartfelt gratitude to the many people who have helped, directly or indirectly, with this book, especially my Reiki Masters Kristin Bonney and William Lee Rand, who were instrumental in starting me on my fascinating journey with Reiki, and Andy Bowling, Ann Rogers, and Rick Rivard, who taught me the original Usui techniques from the Japanese lineage. In addition I would like to thank the many other Reiki Masters who have inspired or informed me in different ways, including Hiroshi Doi, Frank Arjava Petter, Mari Hall, Light and Adonea, Carol and Mark Melling, Wendy Monks, Rev. Simon-John Barlow, Paula Horan, Walter Lubeck, and others I have met and exchanged views with along the way.

Also I would like to thank the many spiritual teachers and writers who have helped to form my ideas and beliefs, especially Gill Edwards, Deepak Chopra, Caroline Myss, Neale Donald Walsch, Louise L. Hay, Mike Robinson, and others too numerous to mention. In addition I would like to say how grateful I am to all my Reiki students for the love and learning they have brought me, and in particular Adrienne Earp and her father, Gordon Earp, whose cheerful courage and unshakable faith in Reiki and self-healing were truly inspiring during the last few months of her life.

I would also like to express my thanks to my son and daughter, Chris and Kathy Roberts, for their loving support, and of course to the staff at Piatkus and Tarcher for their practical help and advice, and to Rodney Paull for his excellent illustrations.

INTRODUCTION

A Personal Self-healing Journey

Since the early 1990s there has been an explosion of interest in personal health issues, including all forms of healing and complementary therapy, particularly in the West. Reiki has become one of the best-known and most widely practiced healing systems, partly because it is simple to use and quick and easy to learn, and millions of people all over the world have learned how to channel Reiki (a Japanese word meaning "spiritual energy") in order to help themselves and other people.

Self-healing with Reiki is aimed at *everyone* who has Reiki, at any level, whether they have just completed a First Degree course, have practiced their Second Degree skills for a few years or have been teaching Reiki for decades as a Reiki Master, because self-healing is the most important part of Reiki practice. "Healer, Heal Thyself" is a popular mistranslation of Hippocrates' edict "Physician, Heal Thyself," and whatever a person's motivation is when learning Reiki—many people come in to Reiki with the intention of helping others, rather than themselves—it is crucial to use Reiki regularly on yourself both for your own benefit and in order to be better able to help others.

Dr. Mikao Usui, the founder of the healing system that we call Reiki, taught that by healing yourself you also have a healing effect on others, and he referred to his teachings as a "method to achieve personal perfection," with an emphasis on attaining health and happiness. Dr. Usui's teachings were based more on spiritual practice than on hands-on healing, although it did form a part of his system when it was required. Indeed, the ability to perform healing—what was known as *Teate*, the Japanese word meaning "palm healing"—was seen as a by-product of spiritual development, and of minor importance and relevance to the real goal of spiritual development itself.

Usui taught that the most important thing was finding and following one's spiritual path in life, and it was the spiritual path followed by Usui that resulted in the birth of Reiki (see Chapter 1). What Usui eventually did when he began teaching his system in the early 1920s was to give people the tools to heal themselves. In his words, according to one of his original students who is now 106 years old: "You are everything; if you are healing yourself, you heal everything." Usui equated spiritual practice—energy-cleansing techniques, meditation and sensible principles for living a good life—with healing the whole self, body, mind, emotions and spirit, because spiritual development raises a person's energetic vibrations (see Chapter 3) allowing more life-force energy (the "Ki" in Reiki) to flow through them, which has a beneficial effect on their health and overall well-being.

Most people attending their first Reiki workshop (usually called Reiki First Degree, or Reiki 1) are taught that Reiki can be used for self-healing, and they are usually shown the basics of carrying out a self-treatment with Reiki—where to place their hands, and how often and for how long to treat themselves (see Chapter 5). But few discover Reiki's true potential for self-healing, and few are taught the spiritual practices that are the foundation of Usui's original system. Reiki is an amazing tool for healing body, mind, emotions and spirit to create wholeness and harmony, personal peace and a sense of purpose, emotional balance and feelings of joy, bliss and fulfillment. But it helps to know how to use it!

This book is therefore designed to provide access to the real impact and power of self-healing with Reiki, based on my experience of practicing and teaching Reiki, and using it daily on myself for self-healing since 1991. It reveals innovative yet easy-to-use techniques for using Reiki on yourself that will encourage healing on the physical, mental, emotional and spiritual levels, leading to greater self-awareness, self-understanding, personal growth and spiritual development. It also draws on my wide experience of teaching and practicing a range of other metaphysical and spiritual subjects over many years, so it includes special meditations and visualizations, suggestions for improving your surroundings with feng shui, how to use crystals with Reiki and lots more.

Actually writing this book has been a cathartic self-healing experience for me, because as I practiced the various techniques again, and wrote about them, the issues they were designed to heal came to the surface, so I have had what you might call an interesting time! Several times in these past months I have been through what is called a "healing crisis," where symptoms reemerged that I thought I had dealt with, in order for me to heal them at a deeper level. Because like everyone else I am on a healing journey, I would describe myself as a "work in progress." I don't think it would have been possible to write a book on self-healing with any real authenticity if I hadn't experienced some of the health problems, and therefore healing needs, that I have had over the years. As has been the case for many healers, my need for help with my own health, and life in general, is what led me to Reiki in the first place.

Back in the early 1990s when I first encountered Reiki, I was leading a frenetic life as a single parent of two teenagers, working over sixty hours a week in a stressful job as the acting deputy head of a sector in a large college, studying for an Open University degree and trying to have a social life as well. Looking back, I don't know how I did it all. Not surprisingly, I had suffered some periods of ill health, mainly due to stress, so when I came across Reiki and experienced how relaxed it made me feel, it seemed like the answer to a prayer. I couldn't wait to learn how to use it myself, and for the first five years following my Reiki First Degree course in 1991, I was physically in better health than I could ever remember being—I didn't even catch a cold in that time—as I treated myself regularly and practiced Reiki on others in my spare time.

I took my Second Degree course in 1992, and became a Reiki Master in 1994. Throughout that time I continued to live as frantically as before, and in fact by then I had been promoted to a management position in another college, which proved to be even more stressful. By 1997, even with the help of Reiki and regular meditation, I was burned out, and ended up taking extended sick leave due to stress.

This experience gave me the chance to reassess my life, and I eventually chose to retire on the grounds of ill health. I moved to the Lake District in northern England, where I could live a quieter life and give myself the chance to write, which I had always wanted to do. But did I really listen to my body or change the way I lived? Not a bit of it. Instead of downshifting, which had been my intention, I found myself rushing around the country teaching Reiki and other meta-physical courses—literally from the Orkneys in Scotland to London in the south of England—in order to earn a reasonable living.

I hadn't let go of my workaholic ways, so after four months my body tried to call a halt. I suddenly developed rheumatoid arthritis, and of course it was painful and distressing. Despite this, I was so stubbornly entrenched in my workaholic ways that I still tried to carry on, arriving at one Reiki course on crutches. Not exactly the best advertisement for a "healer," I'll admit, but I hate letting people down, so I did what I thought was best for those potential students, rather than what I knew was best for me. So the message from my body got louder.

By the end of the first day of that course I ended up in hospital, and for the next twelve months my arthritis was so bad that I was in and out of the hospital several times, in a wheelchair for much of the time and virtually unable to look after myself because all the joints in my arms, hands, legs and feet were too painful for me to do anything. At times I couldn't even turn the pages of a book because my fingers were so sore, and the pain just went on and on, twenty-four hours a day.

This experience certainly gave me the time to think again. At first all I could think of was to throw everything I knew at my illness to try to get rid of the symptoms—Reiki, affirmations, visualizations and just about anything else anyone suggested. But nothing happened. I didn't get better. And that was the scariest thing. For the previous five or six years, whatever had happened to me—an occasional headache, trapping my finger in a door, spraining my ankle—all I had needed to do was to place my hands on myself and let the Reiki flow, and within minutes, or at the most hours, the pain and swelling had gone. Why wasn't it working now?

I became very depressed, and I asked myself this question many times, but eventually I had to acknowledge that I was ill and accept that at least for the time being, my life would have to be different than it had been because I was unable to do most of the things I used to do. This is when I began to heal myself. As you will see in Chapter 2, there are four stages in the self-healing process, and in my desperation I had found two of them—acknowledgment and acceptance.

When teaching Reiki over the previous few years I had paid lip service to the idea of the underlying causes of ill health, so I knew the theories (see Chapter 2), but when it came to being ill myself I forgot all about it—or probably more honestly, I hadn't wanted to consider it. Now I began to examine this idea, to seek an awareness of why I had become ill (stage three of the self-healing process). By meditating on the issue and seeking guidance from my Higher Self (*see page 205*), I began to realize that I had been abusing my body—and for that matter, my mind, emotional self and spirit—by pushing it beyond its limits of endurance. On both a physical medical level and a metaphysical level, the many years of stress I had subjected myself to had finally caught up with me, and I needed to radically alter my way of life—permanently.

So I took action—the final stage in the self-healing process. I took some simple, practical steps, like changing to a healthier diet and eliminating some foods known to aggravate arthritis, and I changed my attitude to many things, including my resistance to conventional medicines. I had been so fixed in my ideas (interestingly, this is known as one of the causative issues behind arthritis) that I had refused to take anything other than some fairly standard anti-inflammatories and painkillers—and even those only under sufferance.

After I learned to let go of my opposition to everything my doctors advised, lo and behold, within a couple of weeks on a suitable drug I was a different woman! I was mobile again—or at least, mobile enough to get about a bit on crutches, start driving again, cook for myself and generally look after myself. Reiki had finally got through the layers of resistance, and brought to the surface the understanding of the phrase "what you resist, persists." All the effort I had put into resisting my illness had been wasted. All I had really needed to do was to "let go, and let flow."

I gave up trying to live my "old" life, and stopped chafing at the bit and feeling resentful because I could no longer rush around "doing" things; instead I got on with my "new" life—just being me. I don't mean being me in one of the many roles I used to rush around playing—mother, daughter, teacher, business manager, healer, Reiki Master—because they were all masks. For a few years I gave up the life roles other people wanted me to play, and just concentrated on myself.

I ate healthily, slept a lot, gave myself lots of Reiki, meditated regularly, received guidance from my Higher Self, read prodigiously to learn more about myself and my favorite metaphysical subjects, relaxed and generally enjoyed my more peaceful lifestyle—and I allowed my creative self some room so that I could write my first book on Reiki, which was published in 1999.

Since then my health has continued to improve: I am not yet 100 percent healthy, although I have periods when I'm almost there. As I said, I'm still on a healing journey. But now my attitude is that that's OK. There are still lessons to be learned, and sometimes I get a flare-up of the arthritis (which is what happened when I was writing one of the chapters in this book), but it is always because there is some-thing I'm not paying attention to, or because there are some deeper layers of negativity or blockage that need to be released. As soon as I seek an awareness and understanding of the problem, and take action to put it right, the symptoms die down and I'm fine again.

As an analogy, it's rather like a smoke alarm that goes off to keep you safe by warning you that there's a fire; similarly, my body goes off (or flares up) to warn me that I'm going off track in some way. It's my body's personal safety feature. Each of us has at least one such safety feature—one area of our body that "acts up" regularly, such as a tendency to frequent headaches, indigestion, throat infections, skin problems or a bad back. As you'll see in Chapter 2, one of the consequences of increased spiritual development is an increased ability to be aware of such messages from your body, and drawing more and more Reiki into yourself over a period of time will gradually enable you to heal not only the physical symptoms, but also the mental, emotional and spiritual causes of those symptoms.

My life now is totally different than it once was, and Reiki has brought me all those things I have already suggested it could: wholeness and harmony, personal peace and a sense of purpose, emotional balance and feelings of joy, bliss and fulfillment. I cannot imagine life without it. Teaching Reiki has brought me so much pleasure and satisfaction, and I just love having the chance to play a part in the way that Reiki changes people. I really enjoy the amazement on their faces as they feel Reiki flowing through them for the first time.

I know that a major part of my life purpose is to continue teaching and writing about Reiki, and I am excited about the future possibilities. I have recently set up my own Quest Center, where I can teach Reiki and other metaphysical and spiritual courses, and I am doing this at a time in my life when many other people would be looking forward to retirement. But I am now living what I love, and who would want to retire from that?

What I hope I have done by writing this, my third book on Reiki, is to provide you with some unique methods of using Reiki more creatively for your own healing, and for personal or spiritual development. The emphasis here is on enjoying Reiki and having fun using it to help yourself to live a healthier and more balanced life, while at the same time treating it with the respect it deserves as one of the world's greatest gifts—a healing system for anyone and everyone that is easy to learn and easy to use. I wish you joy on your healing journey!

part one

REIKI, HEALTH AND HEALING

chapter 1

REIKI AND HEALTH

Good health is something we would all like to have, and at some times in our lives we do feel wonderfully healthy, but unfortunately at other times we do not. Perhaps perfect health 100 percent of the time isn't possible, because we don't live in a perfect world where everyone has perfect genes, eats a really healthy diet and is brought up in a perfectly balanced, caring, loving environment of harmony, peace, love and joy. Utopia doesn't exist yet! However, *optimum* health is possible. We can make the most of our chances for good health, and as the rest of this book will show you, Reiki is one of the tools we can use to help us achieve it.

WHAT IS REIKI?

Reiki is a Japanese word meaning "spiritual energy" or "universal life-force energy," and in Japan it is used to describe any form of healing that uses spiritual energy.

Reiki is represented in the Japanese Kanji (Japanese alphabet) calligraphy in two slightly different ways. The image on the left is the more modern form, while that on the right is an older and more traditional way of writing the word Reiki.

In the West, the word "Reiki" has become synonymous with one particular system of healing originated by a Japanese Buddhist priest

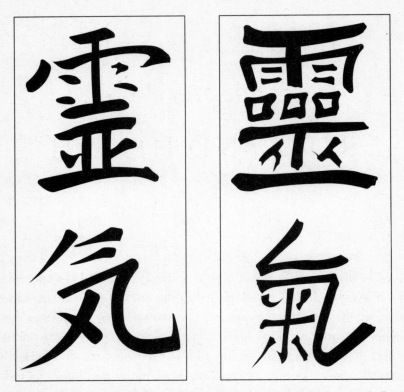

The modern Japanese Kanji for "Reiki": Rei (top symbol) Ki (bottom symbol).
On the right is the older Kanji for "Reiki."

called Mikao Usui (1865–1926), who discovered a way of using spiritual energy to encourage healing of body, mind, emotions and spirit. This became known as Usui Reiki Ryoho, meaning the Usui Spiritual Energy Healing Method.

Usui's system of healing is a safe, gentle, nonintrusive healing technique where Reiki—spiritual energy—flows through a person's hands, which are placed and normally held still in specific positions on the head and body either on the person themselves, or on other people or animals. There is no pressure, manipulation or massage, and as the energy flows into the recipient it helps to balance, heal and harmonize all aspects of the person—body, mind, emotions and spirit. However, the Usui Reiki Ryoho is more than just a form of holistic therapy, as one of its fundamental purposes is to encourage personal and spiritual awareness and growth.

THE DISCOVERY OF REIKI

Dr. Usui began his Buddhist studies as a small child. He eventually explored a number of different forms of Buddhism, traveling extensively, and learning several languages so that he could dedicate many years of his life to the study of Buddhism and other texts on spirituality and healing. In addition to his knowledge of Buddhism, he was an expert in a variety of martial arts, so he had a well-developed understanding of Ki, the life-force energy that permeates all living things.

Although Dr. Usui's major interest was in spiritual development, he did become interested in physical healing, an aspect of Buddhist teachings that had largely disappeared in Japan, where the focus over many centuries had been to purify and heal the spirit rather than the body. When he was in his midfifties, Usui had a profound experience of enlightenment on Mount Kurama in Japan, during which it is said that he received visions of a number of the sacred symbols he had found during his studies, as well as both the gift of healing and the understanding of how to transfer this gift to others. Shortly afterward he developed his healing system, the Usui Reiki Ryoho, which he began practicing and teaching at the clinic he opened in Harajuku, Tokyo, in April 1922.

Although physical healing was an important part of Usui's work—for example, he and his students were acknowledged and thanked by the Japanese emperor for their active involvement in helping the wounded after the Tokyo earthquake in 1923—he also emphasized the necessity for spiritual development, and the Usui Reiki Ryoho incorporated meditation and energy-cleansing techniques, as well as hand placements on the body to allow Reiki to flow to promote healing of physical conditions. In addition, Usui taught five principles for living a good life that he adopted from Emperor Mutsuhito, the Meiji emperor in Japan. Below is a version of these principles that comes from an original document written by one of Dr. Usui's students.

Kyo dake wa	**Just today**
1. *Okoru-na*	1. Don't get angry
2. *Shinpai suna*	2. Don't worry
3. *Kansha shite*	3. Show appreciation (or be grateful)
4. *Goo hage me*	4. Work hard (on yourself)
5. *Hito ni shinsetsu ni*	5. Be kind to others

Mikao Usui is believed to have founded the Usui Reiki Ryoho Gakkai (meaning the Usui Reiki Healing Method Learning Society) in 1926. This is an organization dedicated to keeping the Reiki teachings alive, and the Gakkai members in Japan still follow Usui's teachings very closely. They are fortunate to have in their possession two manuals produced by Usui (the *Usui Reiki Hikkei*); one of these is an explanation of his energy-healing method, the *Usui Reiki Ryoho*, and the other gives details of the various healing techniques he used, including specific hand positions for different diseases and physical problems.

Dr. Usui's system of using spiritual energy for healing is still taught in Japan by some of the more senior members of the Gakkai who have themselves acquired sufficient knowledge and experience of Reiki to be able to teach it. Reiki is taught in three levels, Shoden (meaning "the entrance"), Okuden (meaning "the deep inside") and Shinpiden (meaning "the mystery" or "secret teachings").

It appears that although Usui only taught his healing system for the last four years before his death at the age of sixty on March 9, 1926, in that time several thousand people acquired Shoden from him. Between thirty and fifty people acquired Okuden, but only seventeen reached the highest level, Shinpiden, and these included five Buddhist nuns, four naval officers and eight other men. It seems that not all of the seventeen passed on his teachings, although three of them succeeded each other as presidents of the Gakkai, so enabling Reiki to continue, as he hoped it would. A memorial to Mikao Usui at the Seihoji Temple on Mount Kurama states: "If Reiki can be spread throughout the world it will touch the human heart and the morals of society. It will be helpful for many people, not only healing disease, but the Earth as a whole."

THE DEVELOPMENT OF REIKI IN THE WEST

So if Reiki originated in Japan, how did it come to be so widely known and practiced in the West? The answer to this lies in the fact that one of Usui's Shinpiden students, Chujiro Hayashi, passed on the first two levels of the teachings to a Hawaiian woman of Japanese parentage, Mrs. Hawayo Takata, who was taken ill while visiting her parents, who had returned to live in Japan. She was diagnosed with a tumor and was awaiting an operation for its removal, but instead she had a sudden insight that there was another way to be healed and visited Hayashi's clinic, where she received daily Reiki treatments until the tumor completely disappeared. She was so entranced with Reiki that she begged to learn how to use it, and lived with Hayashi's family and worked without pay in his clinic for about a year in exchange for the first two levels of the teachings. After she had returned to Hawaii and opened a Reiki clinic there, Hayashi and his family visited her, and in 1938 he completed the teachings so that as Shinpiden, she could teach others.

For many years Mrs. Takata was the only teacher of the Usui Reiki healing system in the West; eventually, she taught Reiki in the United States and Canada. Until the early 1970s she taught only the first two levels, Shoden, which she called First Degree, and Okuden, which she called Second Degree. In 1972 she began to teach the Shinpiden level, which she called Third Degree or Reiki Master, and over the next eight years, before her death in 1980, she taught twenty-two Shinpiden students. It is through these twenty-two Reiki Masters and their students that Reiki has spread throughout the Western world.

THE LINEAGE SYSTEM OF KNOWLEDGE TRANSFERENCE IN REIKI

In the above sections I have referred to Dr. Usui, Chujiro Hayashi and Mrs. Takata "teaching" Usui's system of healing, but Reiki cannot be "learned" in any of the ways with which we in the West are familiar. It doesn't actually require any *learning*, in the traditional sense, because it

7

is not knowledge-based—it is experience-based. Being able to use Reiki requires that you channel or draw the healing energy into yourself, and you cannot *acquire the ability* to channel Reiki by reading this or any other book, or attending a lecture, or watching a television program, video or DVD. You can, however, learn *how to use* Reiki through these mediums—for instance, they can show you where to place your hands when carrying out a Reiki treatment.

The ability to channel Reiki energy is passed on from a Reiki Master to a student through a lineage system, which simply means that each Reiki Master can trace their lineage back to the founder of Reiki Ryoho, Mikao Usui—the lineage system is rather like a family tree. As an example of "lineage" within Reiki, I have received initiations and teachings from four different Reiki Masters, two from a Western lineage, and two from a Japanese lineage. My two Western Masters, Kristin Bonney and William Rand, can each trace their lineage through the familiar Western route back to Hawayo Takata, who brought Reiki to the West, and on to Chujiro Hayashi, who was taught by Dr. Usui. However, my Japanese lineage through Andy Bowling and Rick Rivard begins with Kan'ichi Taketomi, another of Usui's Shinpiden (Master) students, and then goes through Kimiko Koyama, a former president of the Usui Reiki Ryoho Gakkai, to Hiroshi Doi, the only Japanese Reiki Master to bring the Eastern lineage Reiki teachings to the West.

This lineage system is important because of the manner in which Reiki is passed from Master to student—by means of a spiritual empowerment that we call an "attunement." In Buddhism a spiritual empowerment is a familiar but very special element in spiritual practice, where energy, existential knowledge, insight and ability are passed from a sensei (respected teacher) by thought and intention deep into a student's mind, body and spirit, and it usually takes place as part of a sacred ceremony.

You may remember that Dr. Usui experienced a powerful enlightenment experience on Mount Kurama, when he received a spiritual empowerment that gave him a deep knowledge and understanding of the Reiki symbols, and the ability to heal (*see page 5*). The spiritual empowerments that are carried out by a Reiki Master in Reiki classes today are similar in nature, but less powerful, since Dr. Usui received the whole understanding and the full strength of Reiki in one single empowerment, directly from the Source (or God, or All-That-Is), which also allowed him to achieve *satori*, meaning "spiritual enlightenment." As Usui had by that time been involved in spiritual and energy practices as a Buddhist and a martial arts expert for about fifty years, he was no doubt energetically well prepared for such a tremendous experience and for the vast amount of healing energy that was passed to him!

BECOMING "ATTUNED" TO REIKI

Within the Reiki community we usually call spiritual empowerments initiations or attunements, as they "initiate" the student into a new life with Reiki ("initiate" means "to begin") and "attune" the student to the unique energetic vibrations of the Reiki spiritual healing energy ("attune" means "to bring into harmony with"). In Usui Reiki there are a number of these spiritual empowerments spread out between the various levels, so that the student has time to "acclimatize" to the levels of energy involved—between one and four attunements at First Degree, one or two attunements at Second Degree, and one or two attunements at Reiki Master level.

The first attunement activates an energetic channel in the student, through which the Reiki energy can flow from the Source, through the student's Soul energy and into their crown chakra (an energy center located at the top of the head), and then through the energy body (the aura, the other chakras and energy pathways called meridians—see Chapter 3 for a full explanation) and out through the hands. Any additional attunements, at either the same or different levels, further expand this energetic channel, increasing the amount of Reiki that can flow through it. It is the attunement process, or spiritual empowerment, which makes Reiki unique, and that allows the ability to heal to be developed so quickly yet so permanently; once you have been attuned you are able to use Reiki for the rest of your life—the ability to channel Reiki never wears off or wears out.

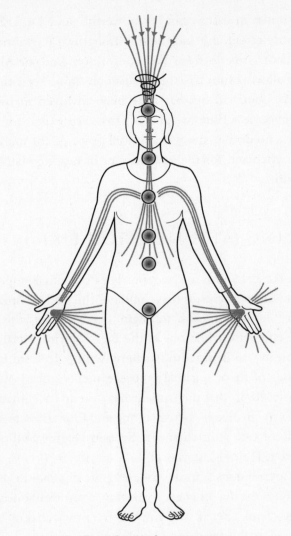

The flow of Reiki after attunement.

Actually, the attunement involves "reopening" or strengthening an existing channel to our enlightened selves (our Soul/Spirit/Higher Self), that part of us which is always and completely connected to the Source/God/All-That-Is. Most people believe that as the Reiki energy enters them through their crown chakra, it must come from outside themselves—from God, or the Universe, or the Source, or whatever term they feel comfortable with. In essence this is true: Reiki does indeed come from the Source. But I believe we have slightly misinterpreted the way in which we access this divine energy, and it only *seems* external because as human beings living in physical bodies we have a limited awareness of our whole existence, and cannot "see" the full extent and potential of our being, our Soul/Spirit/Higher Self and our eternal connectedness to the Divine Source.

The "spiritual empowerment" that takes place during the attunement is just that—it empowers a part of our spirit—Reiki—which we did not consciously know how to access before, so that we become aware of it for the first time and can begin to use it. Once a person has been "attuned" to Reiki in this way, they will always be able to access it easily and simply by just *intending* to use it for self-healing or for healing others. There are no complicated rituals to follow. Energy follows thought, so simply thinking that you want to use Reiki is what "switches it on."

Drawing into our physical bodies more energy of a very high energetic vibration from our Soul/Spirit/Higher Self raises our consciousness and starts a process that continues throughout life—a process of slowly raising awareness of our life purpose, of what we are here to achieve, and how we can achieve it. This is working on a very subtle level, and many people who use Reiki, particularly those who don't use it regularly, or those who are only interested in its physical healing capabilities, are unaware of it. But Reiki works as a catalyst for change, bringing to the surface those aspects of life that are blocking our spiritual progress. Sometimes this can seem a challenging process, but it is always beneficial, as Reiki is divinely guided and always works for our highest and greatest good.

REIKI TODAY

Dr. Usui's system of spiritual energy healing is now used in almost every country around the world, and many other similar forms of healing derived from his original method have been developed in recent years. The main elements of Reiki today are the methods of training, the methods for treatment of oneself and others, the Reiki symbols that activate the healing energy in different ways, and the meditation and energy-cleansing techniques used to complete the system.

Everyone has the innate ability to draw their Soul energy into themselves for healing. Some people develop this skill quite naturally at an early age, while others attend courses for a year or more with organizations such as the National Federation of Spiritual Healers in the UK to learn how to become "spiritual healers." However, the Usui Reiki Ryoho system is probably the simplest and easiest holistic healing method available, allowing anyone to learn to use Reiki in just a day or two, whatever their age or gender, religion or origin. No specific knowledge or previous experience is required; just a desire to learn, a willingness to let the healing energy flow through you, and a little time to attend your first workshop (Shoden/Reiki First Degree), where you take part in a sacred ceremony and receive the spiritual empowerment(s) that then allow the Reiki to flow through you. The way Reiki is taught today in the West does vary from Master to Master, but it is usually taught in three levels, and some Masters will insist on specific time periods and practice between the levels, while others will allow you to progress more quickly.

1. **The First Degree, or Reiki 1**, is normally a one- or two-day course where you receive either a single integrated attunement, or four separate attunements, to open up your inner healing channel and allow the Reiki healing energy to flow through you. The emphasis at this level is on self-healing, so you will be shown how to give yourself a Reiki treatment (*see page 84*), although you will also usually be taught how to carry out a treatment on others, so that you can help your family, friends and pets. You would not normally be advised to practice professionally at this stage, although it is possible to do so (it can, however, be difficult to get professional insurance).

2. **The Second Degree, or Reiki 2**, is generally regarded as the level you need in order to set up as a Reiki practitioner, although many people decide to progress to this level because of the additional scope it gives them for personal healing and spiritual

development. It is usually a one- or two-day course, and it includes one or two attunements that enable you to access even more Reiki. You also learn how to draw three sacred symbols—the Power Symbol, the Harmony Symbol and the Distant Symbol. These are calligraphic shapes that come from ancient Sanskrit and Japanese sacred documents, and you are taught how to use them and their mantras (sacred names) with Reiki. The techniques taught at this level usually include a form of distant healing that enables you to "send" a Reiki treatment to anyone, anywhere, at any time, with the same effectiveness as if that person was with you receiving a "hands-on" healing treatment. You may be required to provide evidence of practice (case studies) before being awarded your Reiki 2 certificate.

3. **The Third Degree, or Reiki 3**, is the level of a Reiki Master (Teacher), and this level may be taught as a whole, or divided into several parts. The training can vary considerably, from a one-, two- or three-day workshop, to a residential course lasting a week or more, and sometimes it is taught like an apprenticeship, in which case a student works alongside a qualified Master for about a year. This level includes one or two attunements, and you are taught the Usui Master Symbol and sometimes two other symbols from Tibet which are not part of Usui's original system. You are also shown how to perform attunements so that you can pass on the teachings to others. This level should be regarded as much more than gaining an extra qualification or some additional skills, because it really means making a lifelong commitment to the mastery of Reiki. (The term "Reiki Master" was a rough translation of *Sensei*, meaning "respected teacher." In reality, no one can "master" Reiki, because it is a divine energy, so in essence being a "Reiki Master" means following a spiritual path toward self-mastery; this can be a physically, mentally, emotionally and spiritually demanding healing journey, although of course it can also be very rewarding.)

When someone has acquired the ability to channel Reiki they are able to carry out Reiki treatments, either informally on friends and family,

13

or formally, as a Reiki practitioner (with Reiki 2 recommended for this). A Reiki treatment takes about an hour, and is usually carried out with the recipient lying comfortably on a therapy couch or a massage table, covered with a soft blanket, or sometimes sitting in a chair. The recipient remains fully clothed (except for their shoes), and the practitioner's hands are placed and normally held flat and still in specific positions over the recipient's head and body. There is no pressure, manipulation or massage, although occasionally there may be some gentle tapping with the fingertips at suitable sites. (No intimate parts of the body need to be touched at any time during the treatment.)

During the treatment the recipient usually feels very relaxed, warm and peaceful as the energy flows through them, although sometimes they might feel tingly or quite emotional as the Reiki brings to the surface old issues and patterns to be released. Some people feel super-energized immediately after a treatment, while others feel very tranquil and sleepy. The person giving the Reiki usually feels good during and after the treatment, too, because they also receive some healing energy while it is flowing through them.

One of the great advantages of being able to channel Reiki is that you can treat yourself. A full self-treatment involves twelve or more hand positions on your head and body, but you can also give yourself Reiki at almost any time—while watching television, for example— by simply placing your hands on any part of your body. Using Reiki on yourself every day is an excellent way to help yourself to relax, and as you will see in later chapters, it can have beneficial effects on all aspects of your health. Self-treatment can also be part of the more spiritual aspects of Reiki, because it can provide a peaceful and meditative experience, especially when it is combined with other Reiki techniques for meditating and cleansing yourself of negative energies (see Chapter 4).

LINKING REIKI WITH HEALTH

For at least 2,500 years, and probably for very much longer, the laying on of hands has been seen as advantageous to someone's health, and there have been "spiritual healers" in many cultures around the world throughout history. In the fifth century B.C., Hippocrates, the father of modern medicine, stated:

> It is believed by experienced doctors that the heat which oozes out of the hand, on being applied to the sick, is highly salutary. It has often appeared, while I have been soothing my patients, as if there was a singular property in my hands to pull and draw away from the affected parts aches and diverse impurities, by laying my hand upon the place, and extending my fingers toward it. Thus it is known to some of the learned that health may be implanted in the sick by certain gestures, and by contact, as some diseases may be communicated from one to another.

Hippocrates was probably referring in general to spiritual healing, rather than specifically to what we call Reiki, but the similarities are obvious.

As I mentioned in the first paragraph of this chapter, perfect health is a fairly idealistic, even Utopian, aim. *Optimum* health, however, is different. Optimum health is achievable. It means making the best of what you've got, and giving yourself the best possible chances by living a healthy lifestyle and nurturing your whole self—body, mind, emotions and spirit. In the next chapter we look at the links between health and healing, and at how Reiki can help your healing processes by influencing all areas of your life, from your physical fitness to your mental, emotional and spiritual well-being.

chapter 2

ALL HEALING IS SELF-HEALING

What is self-healing? It is anything you do to help yourself to achieve wholeness, harmony and balance, whether that encourages better health in your physical body, or an improvement in your mental, emotional or spiritual state, or in your life in general. Most of us engage in some self-healing activities as part of our normal lives; this is a form of self-protection necessary for our survival, although we may not think of it in those terms. Taking a holiday from a stressful job for a week or two, having a long soak in a scented bath, spending an afternoon gardening, deciding to cut down your intake of sugary foods or just taking a breather with a cup of tea away from the children for ten minutes can all count as self-healing activities. So self-healing can occur quite naturally, and it doesn't have to be complicated.

Most of us recognize that ideally we need far more self-healing than we actually currently carry out—which is probably why you are reading this book right now. Obviously, the focus of the book is using Reiki for your self-healing, but you will also find other ideas for self-healing activities, so whether you have already done a Reiki course or not, there will be some things that you can try out as a start on a self-healing regimen to help yourself to better health and greater well-being.

DEFINITIONS OF HEALTH AND HEALING

When we talk about health what do we really mean? Being fit and well? Being free from illness or disease? Are we thinking only of our physical well-being, or do we include our psychological, emotional and spiritual health as well? In the dictionary, "health" is usually defined as "the state of being bodily and mentally vigorous and free from disease," and in 1958 the World Health Organization gave the following definition: "Health is a state of complete physical, mental and social well-being, not merely the absence of disease."

As I mentioned in Chapter 1, perfect health is a very idealistic, even Utopian, aim, which would require a set of improbable conditions, from being born to perfectly healthy and genetically sound parents, to being brought up in absolutely perfect physical, nutritional, environmental, social, emotional, psychological and educational conditions. *Optimum* health, however, is an achievable goal. It means making the best of what you've got, and giving yourself the best possible chances by living a healthy lifestyle and nurturing your whole self—body, mind, emotions and spirit. However let's concentrate for a moment on physical health, and the healing process that helps us to maintain our health.

Healing is described in the dictionary as "to be restored to health; to repair by natural processes, as by scar formation; to cure," but the origins of the word itself are "making whole." On a purely physical level, our bodies have an amazingly sophisticated and intelligent set of healing processes to repair and maintain themselves, from our vital organs to our bones, muscles and skin.

THE PHYSICAL HEALING PROCESS

As an example of the fantastic way in which our bodies repair themselves, let's look at something that can happen to anyone—accidentally cutting yourself while chopping vegetables or brushing against a sharp surface, for instance. Provided you are in a fairly normal state of health (that is, you don't have a condition which

17

could cause possible complications), as soon as blood vessels are damaged around the wound blood is released, but then the blood-clotting mechanism is triggered so that you don't just continue to bleed. If, however, there is substantial blood loss, other mechanisms in your body rapidly restore blood pressure and volume so that your heart can continue to function normally.

As the clotting blood dries it forms a scab, which helps to limit the possibility of bacterial infection, but other protective mechanisms also come into play as white blood cells and other types of cell arrive at the scene and begin to digest dead cells and bacteria. After a few hours, tissue regeneration begins as blood platelet cells release a protein that stimulates cell division, enabling the various types of cell required to be produced quickly wherever necessary, for example contractile cells that form around the edges of the wound, so drawing the regenerating skin tissue inward to cover the wound.

Epidermal cells then migrate to the wound point, and within forty-eight hours the surface will already be covered with a thin layer of skin which, if treated carefully, will keep the wound closed. Over the next week or so further layers will be built up until the cut is completely closed. However, this process tends to produce scar tissue which is coarser than normal skin, so over the next two to four weeks the last stage of the wound-healing process will allow for some restitution and remodeling, so that the final state of the healed cut will be as near to the original structure of the skin as possible.

Fantastic, isn't it? All of that goes on without any conscious effort from you, and apart from possible medical intervention in the form of cleaning the wound, putting in some stitches if it is serious enough to need them, and maybe covering the wound with a bandage or Band-Aid—that's all there is to it.

The Regeneration Process

The above process is just an accelerated version of what goes on all the time in our bodies as cells that are lost through wear and tear are continuously replaced by cell growth and division. There are some parts of us which, it has been believed, don't repair themselves in this way once we reach adulthood, notably the brain and the nervous system, but new research has shown that even these cells can replicate, given certain conditions. However, 98 percent of the cells in your body are replaced in a year—so in effect you have virtually a new body each birthday! Your bone cells take about three months to regenerate your skeleton, although the calcium in the bone takes longer (about a year); your liver gradually replaces itself roughly every six weeks; your skin is renewed monthly, your stomach lining every four days.

Of course, many things can impact on your body's natural healing ability: whether you eat a healthy, balanced diet; whether you drink plenty of water; whether you are too tired or under a great deal of stress; your age and general state of health, and so on. For example, poor nutrition reduces healing rates and increases susceptibility to infection, which further delays healing, and studies have also proved that psychological stress has a similar delaying effect on the body's healing processes.

ALL HEALING IS SELF-HEALING

From the above information you can see that good health isn't just something that occurs automatically, regardless of what you do, and healing isn't something that happens "out there," something which someone else "does" to you. No matter who you visit to help you with your healing, whether it be a doctor, nurse or complementary therapist, and no matter what interventions they might suggest, from medicines to herbal remedies, surgery to massage, there is really only one "healer" of your body, and that is *you*. Your body possesses the mechanisms to heal itself, so all anyone else can do is to help that natural process in some way, whether by conventional, complementary or alternative means.

Of course, your body copes every day with lots of potential hazards. For instance, if it is invaded by a virus such as the common cold, your immune system is mobilised and all those rather unpleasant symptoms you experience, such as a high temperature and a runny nose, are actually the effects of your body fighting off the infection, rather than effects of the virus itself. Indeed, taking medication to lower your temperature when you have a simple cold could be undoing much of your body's good work, because the virus is being killed off by the rise in temperature (although, there are cases where it is essential to bring your temperature down if it gets dangerously high).

WHY AREN'T WE HEALTHY ALL THE TIME?

So if your body is so good at healing itself, why are there times when it doesn't? Why do people continue to suffer from chronic or incurable illnesses? Because healing—and health—are holistic issues, not simply physical ones.

As an example, your body produces cancerous (altered) cells every day, but almost all the time your immune system detects and destroys them. However, if your immune system isn't operating as effectively as it could be, then it is possible that not all the cancerous or precancerous cells will be destroyed. There are several possible reasons for this: perhaps your body is already struggling to fight off another major infection, or your immune system has been seriously affected by some stressful event such as a close bereavement (or even a happy stressful event like a wedding), or your body doesn't have the right nutritional balance to work at optimum strength. Any of these causes, and there are a number of other possibilities, can be at the root of the growth of cancerous cells in an otherwise healthy body.

In many cases even if this happens, providing the immune system can return to normal working capacity fairly quickly, it will tackle any early cancerous or precancerous growth and destroy it, and you will be none the wiser. If the cancer does develop, of course, there are various conventional medical interventions that can help, such as surgery, chemotherapy and radiation treatment. But you have probably also heard of people who have developed mature cancerous growths, yet who have managed to mobilize their own body to destroy the cancer, sometimes with astonishing speed, even without medical intervention.

These people have a very positive attitude and an overwhelming determination to "get better," as well as having supportive and loving people around them. They almost always have a very strong survival instinct and possibly some particular reasons for wanting to go on living, such as family commitments, and they often refuse to believe the prognosis given to them by medical staff, preferring an optimistic view that they can recover, whatever is "wrong" with them. They don't give away their power to so-called medical "experts"; instead, they decide to take a very proactive part in their self-healing, using a variety of techniques—Reiki or spiritual healing, and other complementary therapies and creative visualizations—to help them to trigger their body's own healing ability. Of course, they may also decide to utilize the best that medical science can offer them, giving them the greatest overall potential for recovery. The causes of any serious illness are likely to be complex and multileveled, and sometimes an operation to remove as much as possible of a tumor is vital as the first stage in self-healing.

THE DIFFERENCE BETWEEN HEALING AND CURING

That brings us to another topic—the relationship between healing and curing. Let's start by unraveling some common misconceptions. Many people use the words "healing" and "curing" interchangeably, yet they don't necessarily mean the same thing. *Curing* means completely eradicating an illness or disease, whereas *healing* can occur on many different levels, and doesn't have to be linked with a physical illness at all.

1. **Healing on the PHYSICAL level** This might mean eradicating an illness completely, or it could simply mean limiting or alleviating the symptoms for a time while you learn about and tackle any causative issues on the emotional, mental or spiritual levels.

2. **Healing on the EMOTIONAL level** This could allow you to calm any fears and to reach an acceptance of the effects of the illness, help you to come to terms with loss or bereavement, or allow you to let go of destructive emotions such as anger, jealousy and resentment.

21

3. **Healing on the MENTAL (psychological) level** This could enable you to think differently about your illness, perhaps bringing to your attention the lessons your illness is trying to teach you, and promoting understanding of the causative issues; or it could help you to let go of destructive, negative thought patterns, attitudes or prejudices that are holding you back.

4. **Healing on the SPIRITUAL level** This could enable you to develop a more loving and forgiving relationship with yourself, helping you to achieve greater self-esteem; or it could help you to let go of belief systems that are restricting you, allowing you greater self-expression and creativity; or perhaps even help you at the end of your life to make a peaceful transition into death.

On a physical level, however, let me give you one graphic example to demonstrate the difference there can be between healing and curing. In the case of someone who is unfortunate enough to develop gangrene in their foot or lower leg, it may be necessary to amputate the leg below the knee in order to *cure* the illness—and hopefully, if the disease has been caught in time, the gangrene will indeed be eradicated, and in practical terms the body's natural processes will then be activated to heal the wound caused by the operation.

However, an amputation certainly does not *heal* the person, because such an operation will have an enormous psychological, emotional and even spiritual impact upon them, from the way they view themselves and come to terms with their new body image, to their relationships with other people. Will they still feel loved and attractive, or will they expect or receive rejection from others? What will be the impact on their everyday lives? Can they cope with the challenges to mobility or dexterity that the loss of a limb can cause? What about their future aims, ambitions and potential? Will they learn to live with any restriction and find new outlets for their talents, or will they believe life is simply not worth living any more?

Healing is therefore a very personal thing, but many people still seem to think of it as being healing purely at a physical level, whereas the reality is much wider. Even medical science is at last coming around to an understanding that healing isn't simply a collection of physical processes; it involves the whole person—body, mind, emotions and spirit.

THE BODY/MIND CONNECTION

If you go to a doctor complaining about an upset stomach or painful joints, their trained response is to give you something to deal with the symptom, but to generally pay little or no attention to the actual cause. This may be something purely physical—perhaps you have eaten something that has disagreed with you, or strained a joint through some physical activity—but although those are fairly un-complicated examples, the causes may be more than purely physical.

Knowledge about the way that the mind can affect the body is seen as a fairly recent discovery, but actually most ancient forms of treat-ment, such as Ayurvedic or Chinese medicine, are based on the body/mind connection. Scientists can now explain the connection in a simple way—wherever thought or emotion goes, a chemical goes with it. For example, fear triggers the "fight-or-flight" response and releases the hormone adrenaline; happiness floods the system with endorphins that make us feel good; and endorphins also have the ben-efit of fitting into the body's pain receptors and therefore blocking pain signals to the brain so that we don't feel pain as much as we oth-erwise would.

The understanding that negative mental states get converted into some of the biochemicals that can create disease has helped scientists and doctors to see why chronically depressed people are four times more likely to become ill, why widows are twice as likely to develop breast cancer and why prolonged stress can produce a wide range of physical problems from heart disease to autoimmune system disorders. It has also helped them to realize that positive mental states can have a good effect on health—for instance, cancer patients who have a determination to beat their disease can significantly increase their survival rates.

Moreover, we now know that just getting a patient to *think* that a tablet they are taking will have a beneficial effect will in many cases produce that effect. Many people given a sugar pill, known as a placebo, will for instance experience considerable pain relief, lower blood pressure or even reduced gastric secretions if they have ulcers. Similarly, the side effects of chemotherapy, such as hair loss and nausea, can be produced simply by telling a patient that the placebo they are taking is a powerful chemotherapy drug (although such an experiment seems highly unethical, and probably wouldn't be done in today's medical climate).

From this perspective, it can be clearly demonstrated that the mind can, under some circumstances, control the body. Is it therefore possible that the mind could control the body under *all* circumstances? Could someone produce positive health outcomes purely by using positive intention? This is certainly the view of many people, and not only those who are actively involved in complementary and alternative health practices.

Body/mind exercises including relaxation, meditation and breath control are commonly used to help a variety of physical problems, such as asthma or high blood pressure, as well as mental problems like acute anxiety or panic attacks. Other methods of using the mind to encourage better health include affirmations (positive statements designed to reprogram the way a person thinks or feels about themselves or a situation they are involved in); and NLP (neurolinguistic programming), which consists of a wide range of psychological techniques, again designed to reprogram the way a person thinks and feels, using thought processes, imaging, language and physical "anchoring" of more positive ways of being. It follows that if we could use our minds to help us achieve optimum health, that would be a major step forward, wouldn't it? But how does it work?

BODY WISDOM

There are many people (and I'm one of them) who believe that your body has its own form of consciousness, and that at all times, under all circumstances, your body is trying to be your loving and helpful friend. Every ache or pain, discomfort or disease, illness or imbalance is your body's way of conversing with you. It is always in direct contact with your Higher Self (your Soul or Spirit), in ways in which your conscious mind is not, and your Higher Self, through the medium of your body, uses the solid, physical aspects of yourself to give you messages. Your Higher Self has total, unconditional love for your Whole Self and for your Physical Self, and always wants what is best for you. If you are in some way "off track," or doing things (or even thinking or saying things) that are harmful to you in some way, it uses your body to try to get a message to you—to bring something to your attention. The more "in tune" with your body wisdom you become, the simpler the message is and the faster it is transmitted to you.

Here is an example of how this works. I was invited to a social event recently which was also attended by a couple of acquaintances whom I usually try to avoid because I find their attitudes to be very negative, but on this particular evening the gathering was too small for me to steer clear of them. After about half an hour of general conversation while we were all sitting around the fireside, I was getting really irritated by what they were saying, and found that whenever I turned my head in their direction I would get a sharp pain in my neck. After another few minutes my neck stiffened up so much that I wasn't able to turn in their direction at all!

I quickly began to give myself Reiki to my neck (discreetly, with one hand) and the pain subsided, but for the next hour I had to give myself regular touch-ups of Reiki to keep my neck free to move. Then I suddenly realized what message I had been sent, and smiled to myself—the Reiki had done its work, not only dealing with the discomfort of my physical body, but also allowing the causative factors to rise to the surface of my mental body to be recognized.

Only a few days before I had been on a residential retreat where the focus of the meditations was tolerance and compassion and, as so often seems to happen, I was being "tested" on my learning—in this case, I was found wanting. Once I had recognized the lesson I was being given, and had readjusted my thinking to be more tolerant of my acquaintances' attitudes and more compassionate toward their position, the pain and stiffness went and the rest of the evening was much more pleasant.

I do try to "tune in" to my body, and to understand what is going on, so I often get quick, easy messages like the one I have just described. The most common messages are reactions to negative thoughts or an inability to make a decision and "worrying" over it in my mind. In these cases I tend to get sudden pains in my knee, ankle or foot—all dealing with "where I am going." These are almost always on the left side of my body, which is more directly concerned with my spiritual journey through life than the right side, although if I am thinking negatively about money, or other issues of physical security, then it will be my right leg that reacts.

After my initial reaction of "Ouch!," the stab of pain is enough to make me stop and pay proper attention to whatever I have been thinking about, rather than just letting thoughts idly float around my mind. It directs me to "mindfulness," creating awareness of the present moment, making me pause and just "be" for a while, and allowing me to let my thought processes slow down so that I can eliminate the negativity or indecision. That probably makes it sound easy for me, but it isn't—I'm human, and it can still get me down sometimes, too. I am on my own self-healing journey, just like everyone else, but I feel fortunate to have a belief system that perhaps makes me feel more empowered than some people, and therefore better able to cope with most difficulties.

REACTING TO THE MESSAGES

Most people react to illness or disease by trying to get rid of the symptoms as quickly as possible, usually by seeking medical advice or intervention, and that's a natural enough reaction. No one wants to feel ill. However, a recent advertisement on television caught my attention, because it was extolling the virtues of a popular analgesic as something "for people who don't have time to have headaches." From my perspective this attitude is quite alarming, because while there is nothing wrong in seeking relief for symptoms, if you really want your body to be healed you also need to understand the illness at the causative level, and if you have constant headaches "masking" them with medication and carrying on as if nothing is wrong isn't a long-term solution. You are not listening to what your body is trying to tell you, so although the symptoms might abate briefly they will return because you are not taking your body's advice and acting upon it.

Your first priority is therefore to ask yourself: *WHY am I ill?* From this metaphysical perspective, illness or disease is created by the body—or the body/mind connection—as a helpful message, and as the body is simply a part of our consciousness this means that we actually create our own ill health. There have been many experiments that have shown that the mind can create symptoms such as the ones I referred to earlier. One experiment involved a group of Japanese children who all knew they were allergic to poison ivy. While blind-folded, the children were told that poison ivy was being brushed against their skin—although in fact a totally innocuous plant was being used—and each one almost immediately produced red and blistered skin where the plant had touched them. Their *belief* that the plant would cause a reaction actually caused their body to react as if it was real. So the idea that your mind works with your body to produce illness and disease may be a very challenging concept, but really it is very empowering, because if between them your mind and body have the power to create ill health, then they also have the power to create good health!

TAKING RESPONSIBILITY FOR YOUR WELL-BEING

It is important not to take this on board as some kind of "blame theory." From this perspective you may be responsible for creating an illness at a deep and unconscious body/mind connection level, but this is not being done at a conscious level so there is no blame attached. You therefore should not judge yourself—or anyone else—harshly for being ill. You don't suddenly wake up one morning and say, "Oh, I think I'll break my leg today—that'll stop me rushing around doing too much and I can have a good rest and some time to think about my direction in life!"; or, "Hmm, I've got a lot of suppressed emotion and anger and resentment inside me, so I think I'll let my body develop cancer or heart disease to give me a message I can't ignore." Of course not—from a human perspective that would be utter madness. But from a Soul/Higher Self level the destructive ability of the cancer or the pain of the broken leg are simply experiences on your journey through this physical life. If you heed the messages, all well and good, and you can heal and move on—and if you don't they will lead to different life experiences, so again from the Soul perspective that is still OK. *You are a spiritual being having a physical experience, not a physical being having a spiritual experience.*

I can understand that these theories are pretty difficult to come to terms with if you haven't heard about them before, and they may well challenge your belief system or your concept of how the world works; of course, you are free to take them on board or ignore them— the choice is yours. But if reading about them has sparked at least an interest in finding out more, then there are some recommended books in the Further Reading section (*see pages 263–65*) that you might find useful.

BRINGING SELF-HEALING FROM THE SUBCONSCIOUS INTO THE CONSCIOUS

If all the body's mechanisms can work automatically to heal cuts, bones and more serious illnesses at a subconscious level, how can we stimulate that unconscious activity with our conscious intention? How can we make the body/mind connection work for us?

Unfortunately, it isn't quite as easy as just deciding we want to do it. Activating the positive functions of the body/mind connection takes time, commitment, determination, perseverance and—as this is a book about self-healing and Reiki—a little help from Reiki! We will get to the detail of how to use Reiki on our self-healing in later chapters. First I want to explain the main steps to self-healing that we

28

all need to go through to give ourselves the greatest chance of achieving the kind of health and well-being we all want.

FOUR STEPS TO SELF-HEALING

There are four steps to self-healing: acknowledgment, acceptance, awareness and action.

1. Acknowledgment

The first important stage is to acknowledge that you are in need of healing. Actually, all of us are in need of healing, to a greater or lesser extent, but sometimes it can be hard to acknowledge that not everything is perfect, and that you have a problem. The problem may be a physical one, perhaps a symptom you have been trying to ignore, possibly through fear of what it might indicate. It might be psychological, such as depression, which could be caused by anything from overwork to worries about money. Or it could be emotional, maybe linked to difficulties in a close personal relationship, or feelings of low self-esteem; or spiritual, giving you feelings of hopelessness and despair. It may seem easier to bury the problem so that it doesn't appear to be a problem anymore, and most of us are quite good at doing that. But if we try to ignore problems or push them below the surface, they become blockages at an energetic level (see Chapter 3). Buried problems don't decompose; they just resurface in some other form!

2. Acceptance

The next, and really crucial, stage is to accept that although you might prefer to feel "better," it is actually OK to be where you are now, and how you are now, in terms of physical, mental, emotional or spiritual health. This is often really difficult for people to come to terms with, because it is part of our nature to want everything to be right, to want to feel healthy, happy, calm and at peace with ourselves all the time. But I'm not talking about passive acceptance, or just giving up and not even contemplating life being better. Far from it.

29

I mean a peaceful acceptance, an understanding that everything is as it should be, right now, in this moment, so that whatever restrictions your health problems impose on you are there for a purpose; whatever mental, emotional or spiritual state you are in is where you need to be, at this time. It is an acceptance that all states change, so that your life will change at some point in the future whatever it is like now, because nothing stays the same forever. Everything is in a cycle of constant change. So if the state you are in now is painful or unpleasant, sad or depressing, it will change, and the likelihood is that it will change for the better. You can just "let go, and let God"—a popular phrase which means accepting the way things are now, and leaving the solution up to God (or the Universe or any other phrase you feel comfortable with) to sort out.

Of course, when we are experiencing wonderful, happy, blissful times in our lives, most of us forget that these states don't last forever, either, and that actually most of life tends to be average, mundane or what we call "normal," whatever that is in our terms. So acceptance of life as it is now, in the present, is what the Buddhists call a state of "mindfulness"; in that state, concentrating only on where we are now, and what we are doing now, can be the path to more joy and bliss in our lives, even if those lives aren't exactly the way they used to be.

3. Awareness

The next stage involves developing an awareness of what is at the root of your problem, and this means taking a good look at yourself and everything in your life. What are the main factors that have led up to this problem? How and why has it developed? To get an answer to these questions you might need to read books on metaphysical causes to gain some information, to ask a respected spiritual teacher to help you, to listen to visualization tapes that lead you on an inner journey to discover some of the underlying issues or to meditate to gain insights. But one way or another, the answer lies within. Through any of the ways I have suggested, your Higher Self can guide you to an awareness, but you do have to be willing to listen and learn.

Of course, it's tempting to bury your head in the sand, because developing awareness can be pretty uncomfortable, so beware of just jumping to conclusions, of opting for the first metaphysical cause you read about and saying "that's it." Try to go deeper. What you read in books is meant only to be a guide, something to help you start your search rather than to provide the actual answer. Spend some time thinking about it and meditating on it, and get in touch with how you feel about it. And be brave enough to face up to it, even if you don't like it. Developing awareness of your need for healing can sometimes push you far outside your comfort zone, but your greatest and highest good isn't always served by the easy path. Being honest with yourself is really the best step you can take, even if it is painful sometimes.

4. Action

The final stage is to take action on what you have learned—on what your body wisdom is trying to tell you and what your Higher Self is showing you needs to change. All self-healing is about change. Sometimes it's as simple as eating more healthily or taking more exercise, or making sure you get enough rest and don't burn the candle at both ends. At other times it can be much more complex, and could mean changing your job, moving to live in a more peaceful environment, letting go of a favorite pastime or ending a relationship. It could even be that you need to completely change your life, so that everything from your beliefs and attitudes to your home and working life is just thrown up in the air to see how it lands.

Almost always the change needs to be permanent. If it's about eating healthily, then it's for life, not just for a few weeks until the symptoms subside. If your job has become so stressful that it's destroying your health and/or your home life, leaving it for a few weeks or months by taking sick leave won't be enough. You either need to change your attitude to the job so that it stresses you less, or you need to leave the job altogether. If you've been ignoring your emotional and spiritual needs, and putting up with an abusive or unhappy relationship, taking antidepressants for a few months may calm you down and help you to cope for a while, but they won't solve the problem. Eventually, you will have to find the courage to tackle the situation.

SELF-HEALING IS SELF-LOVING

Human beings are complex creatures, and each of us is completely unique, from our DNA and our fingerprints, to our personalities and perspective on life and the world we live in. Yet despite our uniqueness and individuality, we all have something in common. We all need love, and we all need healing, whoever we are, wherever and however we live, and whatever our state of health. As in the saying "Charity begins at home," love also needs to begin at home—with yourself—and one of the ways in which you can develop and express self-love is with self-healing.

Self-healing is simply caring about yourself; about giving yourself the time and space to be yourself, and at least as much love and attention as you would give to any other person who needed it. Unfortunately, many people find it much easier to care for other people or animals than they do for themselves, yet that is really doing everyone a disservice, because the more we develop a loving relationship with ourselves, the more love we have to give out to others. What comes around, goes around! As Dr. Usui once said: "You are everything. If you are healing yourself you heal everything."

Taking an active part in your own self-healing is a loving act toward yourself. You are showing your body that you love it by being kind, caring and supportive toward it. You are showing your whole self—physical, psychological, emotional and spiritual—that you love it and care about it enough to spend time on it, that you are not just taking it for granted, that you respect it and recognize that it deserves love—that *you* deserve love. Actually, deservingness is a big issue with most people, and is one of the main barriers to self-healing.

Many people will willingly give up hours, days, weeks or even years to care selflessly for someone they love, but are reluctant to give themselves even half an hour a day for some quiet time to themselves—for meditation, giving themselves Reiki, having a relaxing bath with aromatherapy oils or simply being alone with their thoughts. At the root of this reluctance is a feeling that they have to "deserve" good things for themselves. They may be willing to shower others with gifts and time, but never feel good enough about themselves, so of course they never feeling deserving enough, either.

REIKI'S ROLE IN THE SELF-HEALING PROCESS

You will see in later chapters that Reiki can help in all the stages of the self-healing process, whether on a physical level, helping to reduce symptoms, or at the causative levels, psychological, emotional and spiritual. Whatever your motivation for becoming attuned to Reiki, self-healing needs to be your major focus, whether you've just begun your Reiki journey by taking a First Degree course, or have been practicing at Second Degree level for a few years or teaching as a Reiki Master for a decade or more. You have the gift of Reiki primarily for your own benefit, whether you use it for other people as well or not. Dr. Usui's original teachings were really about using spiritual energy, or Reiki, to help you develop spiritually as a way of healing yourself, because by healing yourself you affect others. The ability to use your hands to help other people with their healing was just seen as a useful addition. That is completely opposite to the way in which Reiki has been viewed in the West, where the capacity to help others with hands-on healing has been seen by many as the most important aspect, and the spiritual development of the person channeling the Reiki is either disregarded or seen as merely a beneficial adjunct. Getting back to Usui's fundamental intent for Reiki is, I think, the greatest tribute we can pay to the wonderful healing system he developed and, ultimately, the most valuable thing we can do for ourselves.

part two

ESSENTIALS FOR SELF-HEALING

chapter 3

THE ENERGY CONNECTION

Einstein and later quantum physicists have explained that at the quantum level—which is between 10,000 and 100,000 times smaller than an atom—everything that exists in the Universe is energy, vibrating and oscillating at different rates. Recent studies of quantum physics have led to some fascinating discoveries, although scientists don't necessarily have any firm explanations, just theories. One theory is that all energy exists on a continuum from the most dense and least conscious, or what we call physical matter, to the least dense and most conscious, which we call spiritual energy. Another theory that was first proved experimentally in France in 1982 is that two previously connected quantum particles, separated by vast distances, remain somehow connected. If one particle is changed, the other is also changed, instantaneously—so at the quantum level, all energy is connected.

Why, you may ask, is this of any interest to us in a book about self-healing with Reiki? Because Reiki is a spiritual energy vibrating at a very high rate, and it works at an energetic level both with the physical matter of the body, and with the electromagnetic energy of the energy field that surrounds and interpenetrates the physical body. Learning this helps us to understand why Reiki can aid healing on many different levels, from the physical, to the mental, emotional and spiritual aspects of each individual.

FROM PHYSICAL TO METAPHYSICAL

To explore the energy continuum a little further, let's look at it in rela-
tion to the human body. Our bodies comprise over fifty trillion cells,
yet despite the sophistication and evolution of the human body we
possess no physiological functions that were not already pre-existing in
the biology of a single nucleated cell. Single-celled organisms, such as
the amoeba, possess the equivalents of a digestive system, an excretory
system, a respiratory system, a musculoskeletal system, an immune
system, a reproductive system and a cardiovascular system, among others. Interestingly, while we think of cells as being physical matter, even
though they are too small to be seen with the naked eye most of each
cell is actually space, or rather energy at the quantum level.
Conventional scientific opinion considers the nucleus to be the "command center" of the cell, and as such, the nucleus would represent the
cellular equivalent of the "brain."

Of course, a human baby begins with a single cell which, when
fertilized, begins to divide and increase. During its gestation, an
amazing process occurs where different types of cell begin to form;
cells that can turn into brain cells, blood cells, bone cells, heart cells,
and so on. These cells remember what type of cell they are, and when
they replicate they reproduce not as general cells but as their specific
type. Some theorists describe this as cellular consciousness, meaning
that each cell must "know" and remember what type of cell it is.
Moreover, some theorists believe that all an individual's knowledge,
experience and memories are stored not only in their brain, but in
every cell in their body, which is one idea put forward to explain why
people who receive transplanted organs sometimes develop some of
the likes and dislikes of—and even flashes of memory from—their
organ donor.

From there it isn't too much of a leap back to the body/mind
connection I spoke about in the last chapter, because if each cell
knows everything you have ever thought, said or done, it is hardly sur-
prising that the body can act as a signaling device, giving you "disease"
messages to reflect what is going on in your mind and your life in
general.

If all this is getting too scientific, don't worry—I'm not going to continue in this vein! However, this information will act as a foundation for some of the other theories that will be presented in this and later chapters, so please just bear with me for the moment.

HUMAN ENERGIES

The physical body is something we all know about—we can see it and feel it yet, as I have said, every cell within it is actually energy or light, vibrating at a slow enough rate to make it into visible physical matter. The human body, and the energy field that surrounds and interpenetrates it, is made up of electromagnetic energy, and every person has a unique vibrational energy signature, or frequency, in the same way as we all have unique fingerprints or DNA. We are familiar with the fact that the electromagnetic outputs of various parts of the body—the heart and brain, for example—are detectable by scientific instruments, but the electromagnetic output of a person's whole body can also be measured using an electromyograph. In this connection, some interesting research was carried out on a variety of people a few years ago by Dr. Valerie Hunt, author of *Infinite Mind: The Science of Human Vibrations*.

Dr. Hunt recorded the output at the high-energy sites on the body known as chakras, and some fascinating results were obtained. Most people in the study registered within the normal range, around 250 cps (cycles per second), but when the tests were carried out on people who used healing energies (such as Reiki) and others who actively used their psychic ability, it was found that their frequencies registered in a band between 400 and 800 cps. Even higher frequencies—more than 900 cps—were found in people who were not only healers and psychics, but also followed a very spiritual path, regularly practicing deep meditation.

It therefore seems that drawing more spiritual energy—Reiki—into yourself really does raise the energetic vibrations of your whole body to a higher level; and because the higher the frequency is, the less dense and therefore more conscious the energy will be, it also raises your consciousness, enabling you to become more spiritually aware. I will be expanding on this point later in this chapter, but first I want to describe the energies that are both within the physical body and encircle it.

THE HUMAN ENERGY FIELD

Surrounding and interpenetrating your physical body is another field of energy made up of much finer, lighter and higher vibrations, which is usually called the aura, the auric field or the human energy body. This auric field is as much a part of you as your physical body, but the higher frequencies of the energies that make up the aura mean that it is harder to see it with the naked eye, although it can be detected by some scientific equipment, and a representation of the aura can also be photographed using a special Kirlian camera.

In addition to the aura, our energy field contains some active energy centers known as chakras, and a range of energy channels flowing through the body called meridians, or nadis. Perhaps the easiest way to understand this is to relate it to parts of your physical body. The aura could be described as the energy equivalent of your whole physical body, the chakras could correspond to your brain, heart and other major organs, and the meridians are similar to your veins and arteries, but they carry energy—the life force we call Ki—instead of blood.

The aura is a field of energy or light that completely surrounds the physical body above, below and on all sides. It is made up of seven layers, with the inner layers closest to the physical body composed of the densest energy, and each succeeding layer being of finer and higher vibrations. Most people have an oval (elliptical) aura, which is slightly larger at the back than at the front and fairly narrow at the sides, and stretches above the head and below the feet. Your aura is not always the same size, however. It can expand or contract depending upon a variety of factors, such as how healthy you are, how you are feeling emotionally or psychologically at any given moment or how comfortable you feel with the people in your immediate surroundings.

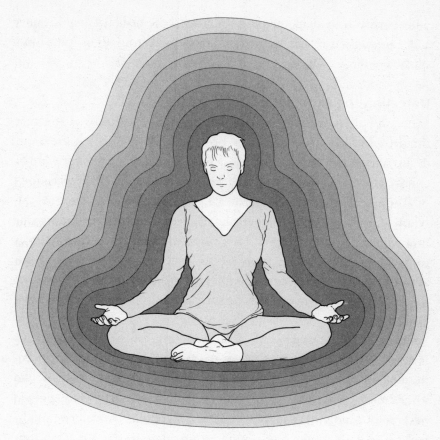

The seven layers of the aura.

The aura is spiritual energy, or life force, or Ki, which is present around each of us from birth (and before birth, as the fetus develops) until around the time of our death. (Usually, just before death only a narrow band of spiritual energy remains, down what is referred to as the Hara line, linking all the chakras in the center of the body; shortly after physical death, no aura can be detected, because the life force no longer exists.) In a living person, the outer edges and the individual layers of the aura can be detected using dowsing rods or a pendulum, and they can also be sensed with the hands. The densest layers, nearest to the body, can also be seen with the naked eye by most people with a little practice, and some very psychic people can see the whole energy body quite clearly. I am sure you will have seen paintings

41

where artists have depicted the aura around the heads of angels, saints and prophets as a bright golden halo, indicating their pure and spiritual energy.

Detecting the Aura

Detecting auras with dowsing rods and with the hands is the first thing I teach in my Reiki classes, because apart from being great fun it also allows people to gain a real understanding of the concept of energy and life force before they learn to use the higher vibrations of Reiki healing energy to permeate, clear, balance and energize the whole energy body. The biggest shock for most people is finding out how large their aura can be! Of course, the size varies from person to person, and it changes from day to day, but the outer layer of the aura can be anywhere from about two meters (six feet) to twenty meters (sixty-six feet) or even further away from a person's physical body.

This means that whenever we are with other people our auras are intermingling, and whether or not we are mindful of it we are "picking up" signals from other people's auras all the time. This is why we sometimes feel a little edgy when standing next to some people because our individual auras are discordant, or alternatively, we might feel particularly drawn to sit beside someone because our vibrations are very harmonious.

You don't need expensive equipment to detect the aura—it can be done with dowsing rods made from old metal coat hangers, or with a pendulum, which can be a crystal or a ring at the end of a fine chain or length of embroidery silk. However, the aura can also be sensed or felt with the hands. The reason for this is that we are all electro-magnetic beings, and as such we are excellent receivers for an enormous range of vibrations of energy—and everything in the Universe is energy, as I have already mentioned (*see page 37*). Everything has a unique vibrational frequency or signature, and if we tune our thoughts into the specific frequency of an object or a particular person, then that is what we find. Just as our *intention* is what switches on the flow of Reiki when we want to use it, our *intention* is all that is needed to "switch on" this innate skill.

The easiest way to sense your own aura is between the palms of your hands. Hold your hands out in front of you with the palms facing each other, about sixty centimeters (two feet) apart, and *intend* to detect your auric energy. Now close your eyes so that you have fewer distractions and can concentrate on any sensations in your hands and fingers, then slowly bring your hands closer together. You may find that your palms get warm, or your fingers begin to tingle, and as your hands get quite close together you may feel a resistance between them, almost as though you have a balloon between your hands. That's your auric energy!

It is also possible to learn to see your aura, and this is accomplished most easily by holding out one or both of your hands in front of you with your fingers spread as wide apart as possible, and then gazing softly at the spaces between the fingers. (You will find it best to have a plain background behind your hand, and to do this exercise in natural daylight.) The innermost layer of the aura is the densest, so this

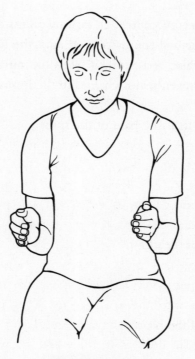

Detecting the aura.

43

is the one most people spot first as a pale bluish, grayish or yellowish mist around each finger, perhaps of a thickness of only one or two centimeters (about a quarter of an inch). With lots of practice you may start to see other soft colors, and occasionally flashes of brighter color.

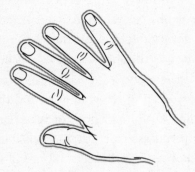

A hand showing an energy field.

THE CHAKRAS

The chakras are energy centers at various points around the energy body where the spiritual energy of your aura, the Ki, or life force, circulates actively. Chakra is a Sanskrit word meaning "wheel" or "vortex," and there are seven major chakras in the human body located at:

1. The perineum, near the base of the spine.

2. Near the navel.

3. At the solar plexus.

4. In the middle of the chest.

5. At the throat.

6. In the center of the brow.

7. On the crown of the head.

In addition, there are a number of minor chakras, for instance in the palms of the hands, on the knees and on the soles of the feet. A healthy chakra vibrates evenly in a circular motion, resembling a funnel that is fairly narrow close to the body, but which becomes wider as it gets further out.

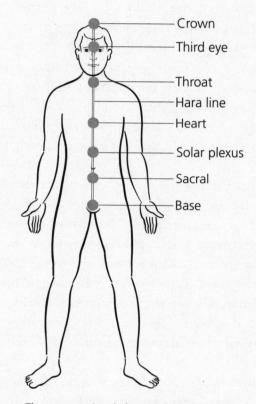

Crown
Third eye
Throat
Hara line
Heart
Solar plexus
Sacral
Base

The seven major chakras and the Hara line.

Detecting Chakras

Many people who practice Reiki find it quite easy to detect and locate each of the chakras when they are scanning their own or someone else's body before a Reiki treatment (see Chapter 5), but you can also use a pendulum. You first need to "tune in" to the vibrations you are seeking—in this case those of the chakras. Hold the pendulum still (this is easiest if your arm is supported) and silently or aloud ask, "What is positive?" and then "What is negative?" For me, the pendulum rotates in a circle in a clockwise direction for positive, and counterclockwise for negative, but you may find that it circles the opposite way, or swings from left to right, for one, and backward and forward for the other. (Note that the terms positive and negative in this connection merely indicate different polarities of energy, as in magnetism, and have nothing to do with good or bad!)

You can detect your own chakras, but to begin with it is easiest to see how this works with someone else. For this exercise it is therefore probably best if you ask a friend or partner to lie down, and then hold the pendulum about five to ten centimeters (two to four inches) above their body. Starting either above the head or above the feet, slowly move the pendulum along an imaginary line running down the center of the body (that is, as if the line runs through the nose and navel).

When you reach the location of a chakra, the pendulum should begin to rotate or swing—rotation is more common because the energy of the chakra is swirling like a vortex, so the pendulum tends to follow the energy. Some chakras may rotate in a clockwise direction, and some in a counterclockwise direction, or they may all appear to be the same. However, you will probably find that if you raise the pendulum to about thirty centimeters (twelve inches) above the body, it will rotate in a wider arc, echoing the funnel shape of the chakra's energy, which is narrower near the body and wider further away from it.

Sometimes the chakra's outer edge is only a few inches from the body, but it can extend up to one meter (three feet) away, depending upon the physical, mental, emotional and spiritual state of the person. A really healthy, balanced and open chakra will make a pendulum swing vigorously, whereas one that is unhealthy, unbalanced or blocked will hardly move the pendulum at all.

Don't panic if when you first start dowsing for chakras the pendulum doesn't move much! This may simply be because you are too tense for your body's electromagnetic energy to flow easily, which can interfere with the accuracy of the result; try to relax your body, especially your shoulders, and it should prove easier. If you try this exercise before and after a Reiki attunement or treatment, you will usually find a greater reaction from the pendulum afterward, as the flow of energy in the chakras becomes more balanced after Reiki.

REIKI AND THE HUMAN ENERGY FIELD

I have briefly mentioned Ki as meaning life-force energy, the energy that flows within the physical body through the chakras and meridians, as well as around the body in the aura. This life force has been acknowledged by many cultures for thousands of years—in China it is called Chi, in India it is Prana, whereas in Japan it is referred to as Ki.

In the East medical practice has long been centered around this life-force energy, and "energy-medicine" treatments such as acupuncture, shiatsu and reflexology all work at this energetic level. This is based on the assumption that our life-force energy is responsive to whatever happens to us, including our thoughts and feelings, and that it can become disrupted, or blocked, if the negative aspects of any actions, thoughts or feelings aren't cleared. These blockages in the energy field can eventually become so dense that they transform from the higher vibrations of the auric field into lower vibrations that then affect the physical matter of the body, becoming illness or disease.

Reiki is an energy of an even higher vibration than our normal life-force energy, so channeling Reiki into ourselves helps to break through these blockages, flowing through the affected parts of the physical body and the aura, charging them with positive energy and raising the vibratory level of the whole energy field. It begins a process of clearing and balancing the chakras and straightening the energy pathways (meridians), allowing the life force to flow in a healthy and natural way around the whole body.

Once the life force can flow fully again, it can begin to release the previously trapped dense and negative energy either through the aura or through the physical body, depending upon the density and/or severity of the blockage. If it expels the negative energy through the physical body, which it tends to do with particularly dense blockages, this can be through the normal excretory system, so you may need to go to the toilet more often; or you may sometimes sweat more, or produce more nasal mucus, or even in extreme cases vomit or have diarrhea—although fortunately, this happens very rarely! If the life force releases the negative energy through the aura, this often feels like a cool breeze, although it can just as easily feel hot, tingly, buzzy or just slightly strange.

SOUL ENERGY

As I have said, bringing more spiritual energy (or more of your own Soul or spirit) into yourself is what you do when you intend to channel Reiki into or through yourself. Reiki is part of your Soul energy, or Higher Self, which is of an even higher and finer vibration than your aura, and it is absolutely pure, loving, wise and totally un-affected by whatever you think, say or do, because it is always directly linked to the Source—or God, the Universe or whatever other term you are happy with. The idea that there is more of you than can fit inside your physical body can be quite difficult for some people to comprehend—although I have already mentioned that your aura can stretch out up to twenty meters (sixty-six feet) or more around you, which may be amazing enough. However I want to try to put that into perspective with your Soul energy, which is truly immense and unlimited. Try this:

1. Imagine standing in a large room. Your aura can easily fill the room.

2. Imagine that you are in the middle of a really huge space such as a theater or sports stadium. Your aura could actually spread out even that far around you if it needed to.

3. Now imagine yourself as just one person surrounded by a huge city like London or New York. Your aura could stretch out for a few blocks, but your Soul energy, or Higher Self, could spread out

beyond the edges of the city. Indeed, it could spread out beyond the edges of the country, or even the whole planet or the whole Universe. It is vast, infinite and eternal. And it is connected to all other Souls, and to the Source, at all times, and throughout time. Quite an image, and probably enough to stretch your imagination for the time being!

I've described your Soul energy in this way to let you see the enormous power and the potential that you have when you access Reiki, because what you are doing is drawing into yourself more of your own spiritual energy—your Soul energy or Higher Self—only a small amount of which normally resides within your physical body and aura. The more you use Reiki and the more often you draw it into yourself for treatments or during meditation, the more of your Higher Self remains within your auric field, which is what raises your energy vibrations. The very high vibrations of your Higher Self help you to become increasingly "enlightened"—that is, lighter than the normally dense physical matter of your body—and this leads to greater spiritual awareness, and to an increasing need for personal growth and spiritual development.

CONSCIOUSNESS

Which brings me to the subject of consciousness. You may remember that I mentioned that the energy continuum spreads from dense physical matter at one end, to spiritual energy or consciousness at the other end (*see page 37*). A metaphysical approach assumes that each person's consciousness is made up of three parts:

1. **The Super-conscious Self, or Higher Self**, which I have just been describing as the part of us that we might call our Soul or spirit. This is our true self, which is fully connected to the God/dess consciousness and has full knowledge of our life purpose and the lessons and experiences we have chosen for this life. It is that very wise part of ourselves which is totally loving and supportive, and

always working with us for our greatest and highest good by subtly guiding us and providing us with intuition and deep insight, whether we choose to acknowledge and act on this wisdom or to ignore it.

2. **The Conscious Self**, sometimes referred to as the Ego, is who we think we are, in other words our thinking, speaking, acting self, our personality, our beliefs, attitudes, concepts, likes, dislikes and so on—everything that makes us recognizable as ourselves. The Conscious Self is not necessarily aware of the helpful insights provided by either the Higher Self or the Subconscious Self, but can operate independently until such time as a person is ready to begin to discover more about themselves.

3. **The Subconscious**, which works with the Higher Self to provide intuition and insight to the Conscious Self through dreams, visualizations, instinctive "feelings" (or "gut reactions") and other aspects of "Body Wisdom" and the body/mind connection.

A SUMMARY OF THE METAPHYSICAL APPROACH

That brings me to a summary of the metaphysical approach, where everything is seen as energy, and all energy is seen as interconnected—and science, in the form of quantum physics, now upholds this viewpoint. From this perspective everything that we call physical or real is energy, and all energy is seen as the product of creative consciousness. Creative consciousness is described as God or Goddess, the Source, All-That-Is or even the Universe, and as everything is connected this means that each of us, every individual, is also a part of that consciousness.

This viewpoint is very empowering but also very challenging, because it sees each of us as cocreators with the Source, actively creating our own reality by using our consciousness, or thoughts and intentions, to attract events, situations and people into our lives. The metaphysical view is that everything that happens to us, everything we experience, has meaning and purpose, so there is no such thing as luck (good or bad), or coincidence. We are therefore not helpless victims of random events, but powerful creators of our lives, using the circumstances we create to help us to develop and grow as people—and as souls.

The world we collectively create—our existence on this planet Earth—reflects the mass consciousness, the overriding beliefs, concepts, attitudes, fears and desires of the majority of people. The world we individually create—what we think, say, do, experience, who we meet and relate to, where we live and so on—reflects our *personal* beliefs, concepts, attitudes, fears and desires. *We are spirits having a human experience, not humans having a spiritual experience.*

This is where self-healing fits in. Self-healing can help us to re-create ourselves physically, mentally, emotionally and spiritually. It puts the power back into our own hands—literally, when we are referring to Reiki! In the remainder of this part of the book you will find practical ways of clearing your energies and treating yourself with Reiki. In later parts there is guidance on specific types of self-healing for your energy body and physical body, as well as your mental, emotional and spiritual self and your whole life. I hope when you begin using these ideas you will find them—literally—life changing!

chapter 4

ENERGETIC PROTECTION AND CLEANSING

Whatever level of Reiki you have—1, 2 or 3—it is really important to include a regular energy-cleansing routine in your self-healing, whether you intend using Reiki on other people or not. As I have explained, everything is energy, and energies can have negative, positive or sometimes neutral vibrations (*see page 46*). Being attuned to Reiki raises your body's vibrations, and as the energetic oscillations become faster this makes your whole energy field lighter and less dense as you gradually become more and more "enlightened." This not only increases your spiritual awareness, which I will be dealing with in later chapters, but also means that your whole energy field can become more permeable and therefore more vulnerable to denser energies, which are attracted to the light.

This happens because as your energies become lighter and vibrate faster, there is more "space" between the energy molecules, which the denser, negative energies attempt to fill. As an analogy, imagine placing pebbles in a bowl until it is full; it appears to be completely filled, but if you poured water into the bowl, the water would occupy the space between the pebbles. It is therefore essential to cleanse your entire energy field regularly, because otherwise it can become clogged with negative energy from outside sources—and if it becomes too blocked this could potentially manifest as illness.

The outside sources of negative energy are many and varied, and they can include physical energy, mental or thought energy, emotional energy and spiritual energy. Newspapers, television, radio and films often have sad, disturbing or horrific images and words that can impact negatively on our energy fields, because we react to them mentally and emotionally. It is therefore important to be discriminating about what you read, watch or listen to. It is far better to be uplifted by beautiful music or happy, fun programs, than to be dragged down by horror films or the negative stuff that is usually presented as "news."

Energy disturbances or blockages in other people's energy fields can also impact on us. They include negative thoughts and emotions, and negative blockages such as physical or mental illness, so our energies can be lowered when we spend time with negative people. Moreover, places can impact on our energies, especially if we spend time somewhere where negative energy can collect, such as shopping centers, city streets, offices and other workplaces, doctors' offices, hospitals and even potentially our own homes or homes belonging to friends and family. A home where there has never been a conflict or argument would be very rare indeed, and the mental and emotional energy from such friction can hang around for quite a long time.

Essentially, your beautiful, sparkling, clear and "enlightened" energy body can act like a sponge, mopping up the negative energy soup around you on a daily basis. Not exactly a happy thought, is it? In this chapter I am providing you with some methods of protecting yourself from negative energies, as well as a range of techniques for clearing and cleansing your whole energy body.

USING ENERGETIC PROTECTION

Protecting yourself energetically doesn't have to be complicated. You can use your thought energy (which is very powerful) to visualize protective barriers around yourself, and of course you can use Reiki, with or without the symbols. A sensible way to use these methods is to carry out one or more of them every morning, especially before leaving home, although you can also use them at any time you feel particularly threatened, for example when you are going into some stressful situation or if you have to deal with very negative people in a work or social situation.

◆ Imagine yourself in a bubble or eggshell of white or golden light that is filled with Reiki, and *intend* that the edges of the bubble are permeable only by love, light, Reiki and positive energies. As a second stage to this method, you can also imagine and *intend* that the bubble is closely surrounded by a fine mesh made of gold, and that this mesh is only permeable by love, light, Reiki and positive energies.

◆ If you ever feel really threatened, then do all of the above, and outside your bubble or eggshell of light filled with Reiki and covered with gold mesh, imagine and *intend* that there is a ring of fire. Outside that imagine and *intend* there is a shiny shell made of mirror or shiny silver or gold, with the mirrored/shiny side facing outward. This effectively forms an energetic boundary around you, so that any negative energy sent your way will rebound back to its source.

◆ If you know the Reiki symbols, draw a Power Symbol on each palm, saying its mantra three times, and then stroke and smooth as much of your aura as possible with your palms (about fifteen centimeters/six inches away from your body), *intending* that the Reiki flows into your aura above, below and on all sides of you, to provide a protective shield against any negative energies.

◆ Another beneficial way of using the Power Symbol is to draw it large in front of you and step into it, saying its mantra three times. Imagine being wrapped inside the Power Symbol, so that it is above, below, in front, behind and on each side of you, and intend that the Reiki protect you from any negativity or harm.

USING ENERGETIC CLEANSING

Since the late 1990s we have known in the West that Dr. Usui used a number of energetic-cleansing methods as part of his healing system, and we start this part of the chapter with the Reiki cleansing techniques from his traditional Japanese lineage. It isn't necessary to use the Reiki symbols when carrying out these methods, so anyone with any level of Reiki can use them, but if you have Second Degree you can enhance the process by drawing a Power Symbol over each hand before you start, *intending* that Reiki should flow to clear and cleanse your energy body.

Gassho

You will see *Gassho* mentioned quite often in this book: the word itself literally means "to place the two palms together," and this is probably the most basic of all the *Mudras*—symbolic hand gestures or positions—used in either Eastern or Western spiritual traditions (in the West we would usually refer to it as the "prayer position"). It is a gesture of respect, humility and reverence, used to help to bring the body, mind and spirit into a state of calmness and oneness with All-That-Is. It can be used to begin and end any of the Reiki techniques in this book, as a sign of prayerful respect and honor of Usui's wonderful healing system, the Reiki energy itself and all creation.

To present a *Gassho*, place both hands together with their palms touching and the fingers and thumbs close together and extended

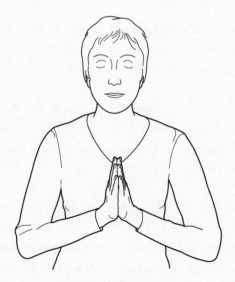

Gassho hand position.

upward in a prayer position, and hold them so that the thumbs are close to the center of the chest, over the heart chakra (*see page 45*). After a few moments, still keeping your hands together, bow slightly as a mark of respect, then move your hands apart again.

The Reiki Shower Technique

This first technique from the Japanese tradition activates and cleanses your whole energy body by flooding it with Reiki like a shower of light, and it is so quick and easy that you can use it almost anywhere. It is ideal first thing in the morning, before a real (water) shower, or before and after a self-treatment, as well as for cleansing yourself at other times of the day—for instance when you've just been with argumentative or negative people, or have just visited someone in hospital.

1. Stand or sit and make yourself comfortable. Close or half-close your eyes and begin to slow down and deepen your breathing until you can maintain a naturally slow and steady pace.

2. Place your hands in the *Gassho* position. Stay like this for a few moments, and *intend* to use Reiki to cleanse and activate your energy body.

3. Separate your hands and lift them above your head, as high as possible, keeping them about twenty to thirty centimeters (eight to twelve inches) apart, but with the palms facing each other.

4. Wait for a few moments until you begin to feel Reiki building up between your hands (as a tingling sensation, or warmth or coolness, for example), then turn your palms downward so that they are facing the crown chakra on the top of your head.

5. Visualize and *intend* that you are receiving a shower of Reiki from the palms of your hands. The Reiki is flowing over and through your whole physical and energy body, cleansing you and removing any negative energy. If you have Second Degree, you can imagine an image of the Power Symbol flowing through you if you wish,

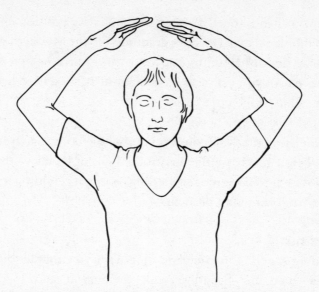

Hold hands above the head, focusing the Reiki to the crown.

and Reiki Masters can visualize the Master Symbol flowing through instead (or as well). Silently say the symbol's mantra three times, imagining it vibrating throughout your energy body.

6. When you feel the vibration of the Reiki energy flowing over and through you, move your hands, palms still facing toward you, and begin to draw them slowly down in front of your face and body, keeping your hands about twenty to thirty centimeters (eight to twelve inches) away from your body. *Intend* that Reiki is flowing from your hands and continuing to cleanse and revitalize you as you draw your hands all the way down your body and then down your legs to your feet. Eventually turn your palms to face the floor and gently throw the energy off your hands so that any negative energy flows out of your feet and into the earth below, *intending* that it be transformed and used by the planet.

7. Repeat this exercise a few times—I find three times to be ideal—and you should feel cleansed, revitalized and more alive as Reiki healing and light flow into all of your cells and fill every part of your body.

8. Place your hands together again in the *Gassho* position and spend a few moments experiencing gratitude for the Reiki, then finish. You may find it helpful to clap your hands once or twice to help you to return to a more wakeful state if this exercise leaves you feeling a bit "spaced out."

After completing the Reiki shower your whole body is activated with Reiki and your hands are filled with the light of Reiki, so this might be an ideal time to do some self-healing—or you can just get on with whatever you planned to do next.

Hatsurei-ho

The *Hatsurei-ho* is a particularly important technique because it combines energetic cleansing with meditation and is therefore excellent for enhancing your Reiki channel and helping you to grow spiritually, as well as for helping to rid your energy body of negative energies. In fact, I would recommend that you make it a regular part of your spiritual practice, as it is an ideal way to start the day or to begin your practice of Reiki, whether treating yourself or other people.

Part of the *Hatsurei-ho*, the *Kenyoku-ho*, is a powerful energy-cleansing technique that cuts through and brushes off negative energies in the energy field, so it can also be done on its own—for example, before taking a shower—then any negative energy can drain away when the water is switched on, to be transformed by the earth. Although the length of the following description may make the *Hatsurei-ho* look complicated, it is actually quite simple. It can take as little as ten minutes, or you can stretch out the more meditative parts of it (*Joshin Kokyu Ho*: the cleansing breath, and *Seishin Toitsu*: concentration or meditation) to half an hour or more—it is up to you.

Kihon Shisei—*Standard Posture*

Make yourself comfortable in a sitting position either on the floor or on a chair, then allow yourself to relax and close your eyes. Focus your attention on your *Tan-dien*, an energy point that is between three and five centimeters (one and two inches) below your navel. With your hands on your lap, palms facing downward, spend a few moments concentrating on bringing your breath into a slow, steady rhythm as you center yourself and focus your thoughts, and *intend* to begin the *Hatsurei-ho*.

Kenyoku-ho—*Dry Bathing or Brushing Off*

The brushing can be done either with contact, touching your body, or more easily without contact about five centimeters (two inches) away from your body, in the aura. Each of the movements is swift and definite. Focus on your breath for this exercise, breathing out as you brush, and making a short, sharp sound as you exhale, such as "haaah."

1. Place the fingers of your right hand at the point where your collarbone meets your left shoulder, with your palm facing the floor, fingers and thumb close together.

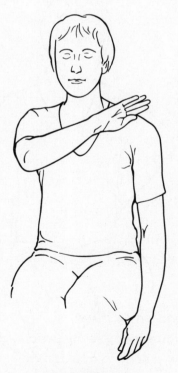

Starting hand position.

2. Draw your hand down with a quick, sweeping movement diagonally across your chest in a straight line, from your left shoulder down to your right hip. At the same time, expel your breath quickly, making a short, sharp sound throughout the movement—for example, "haaah."

3. Now do the same thing on the other side, placing your left hand on your right shoulder, palm facing the floor, fingertips by the collarbone, and brush down from the right shoulder to the left hip, again exhaling loudly.

4. Return to your right hand on your left shoulder and repeat the process again, with your right hand brushing diagonally from your left shoulder to your right hip while exhaling loudly.

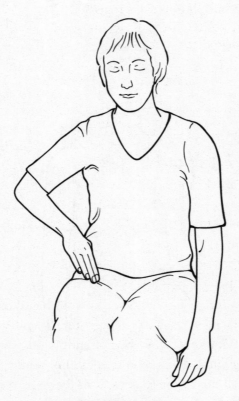

Finished hand position.

(Next you are going to repeat the process, but this time instead of brushing diagonally across your body, you will be brushing along your arms from shoulder to fingertips.)

5. Place your right hand on the edge of your left shoulder, with your palm facing the floor and your fingertips just on the edge of the shoulder.

6. Keeping your left arm straight and at your side, sweep your right hand quickly down the outside of your arm, all the way to the fingertips of your left hand. At the same time, expel your breath quickly and loudly as before, throughout the movement.

7. Repeat this process on the other side, with your left hand on your right shoulder, brushing down quickly to the fingertips of your right hand and expelling your breath loudly.

8. Complete the process by once more sweeping your right hand down your left arm from shoulder to fingertips, again exhaling loudly.

Connecting to Reiki

Now raise both your hands in the air above your head with your palms facing each other about twenty to thirty centimeters (eight to twelve inches) apart, and visualize and feel the light and vibration of Reiki flowing into and between your hands and running through your whole body. When you can sense this vibration, continue with the next section.

Joshin Kokyu Ho—Cleansing Breath

1. Now lower your arms slowly and put your hands on your lap with your palms facing upward; breathe naturally and steadily through your nose. Begin to focus your attention on your Hara line (a major energy line running through the center of your body, connecting all the major chakras from the root to the crown) and allow your body to relax.

2. Concentrate on your breathing. As you breathe in visualize Reiki as white light pouring in through your crown chakra into your Reiki channel and down the Hara line through your major chakras, *intending* that the Reiki cleanse your energies. Then imagine the Reiki spreading out, expanding to fill the whole of your body from your head to your toes and from your shoulders to your fingertips; sense it cleansing and clearing any negative energies from your physical and energy bodies, and feel it melting all your tensions away.

3. As you breathe out, visualize the Reiki light expanding so that it flows through your skin, spreading out to fill your aura. Imagine it flowing beyond your aura in all directions, taking with it any negative energies that have been collecting in your physical or energy body, to be released and transformed by the healing power of Reiki.

4. Continue this process for a few minutes, or as long as you wish, breathing in the cleansing light of Reiki, and letting go of negative energy with each exhalation.

Gassho

Put your hands together (like praying hands) and hold them in front of the center of your chest, a little higher than your heart.

Seishin Toitsu—*Concentration/Meditation*

1. Keeping your hands in the *Gassho* position, take your focus away from breathing through your nose and imagine that you are breathing in Reiki through your hands.

2. As you inhale, visualize the light of Reiki flowing in through your hands, and from there into your heart chakra. Imagine it filling your heart chakra and then sense it flowing into your Hara line. Visualize it flowing up and down your Hara line, connecting all your chakras and energizing them with Reiki, until both your Hara line and your chakras are filled with the white light of Reiki.

3. As you breathe out, visualize the Reiki light from your Hara line radiating out again through your hands, flowing out and spreading Reiki beyond your own aura in all directions, around the world and into the Universe to infinity, spreading peace and healing wherever they are needed.

4. Continue this process for a few minutes or as long as you wish, breathing in Reiki through your hands, into your Hara line and out of your hands again, then let your mind settle into a peaceful, meditative state.

Gokai Sansho

In the traditional way, Japanese Reiki students would now say the Reiki principles aloud three times—obviously in Japanese! You may feel you would like to do the same, either in Japanese or in English; I've given the Japanese phonetic pronunciation in brackets so you can try speaking the words in Japanese if you wish.

Kyo dake wa   Just for today
(*Kee-oh dah-kay wah*)

Okoru-na   Don't get angry
(*Oh-koh-roo nah*)

Shinpai suna   Don't worry
(*Shin-pie soo-nah*)

Kansha shite   Show appreciation (or be grateful)
(*Kan-shah she-tay*)

Goo hage me   Work hard (on yourself)
(*Gyo-ho hah-gay may*)

Kito ni shinsetsu ni   Be kind to others
(*Kee-toe nee shin-set-soo nee*)

Mokunen

Place your hands back onto your lap with the palms facing downward, and *intend* that the *Hatsurei-ho* be completed. When you feel ready, open your eyes and shake your hands gently up and down a few times, to bring you back to a greater state of physical awareness. You are now ready to get on with your day, or to begin your practice of Reiki, either as a self-treatment or the treatment of others.

OTHER TECHNIQUES FOR PERSONAL ENERGETIC CLEANSING

First and Foremost—Cold Showers!

Yes, I know this might be an unpleasant thought, but to cleanse both your physical and energy bodies fully I recommend a cold shower. **If you have any health condition that might make you particularly susceptible to shock from the cold water, ask your doctor before adding this technique to your cleansing routine.**

Cold water is different energetically from hot water, and when its vital cleansing energy flows over your physical body and through your energy field, the "shock" of it shakes loose the negative or "sticky" energy that is trapped in and around your body. Of course, most of us prefer a warm or hot shower for cleaning our physical bodies, and they can also be very relaxing, but energetically they have the effect of expanding your aura, which can potentially make the negative, "sticky" energy enter further into your energy body so that it becomes harder to remove. This is why it is important to *start* your shower with cold water rather than ending with it, although you can do *both* if you wish.

I am not asking you to be a masochist and stand under the shower-head for ages! It is only necessary to let the cold water flow over your chakras, so that they are cleansed, and this can be done quite quickly and easily—the whole process need take no more than fifteen to twenty seconds. If you wish, you can quickly jump under the cold water, and turn around so that the water flows over the crown of your head and down all the front and back chakras, as well as the minor chakras and main meridian points on your shoulders, elbows, wrists, hands, hips, knees, ankles and feet. Then you can turn the water temperature up to what you normally prefer. (You can wear a shower cap if you don't want to get your hair wet, as your crown chakra will still be cleansed by the water flowing over the cap.)

Personally, I find it easiest to hold the showerhead in my hand, so that I feel more in control of where and for how long the cold water showers on to me. Making sure I always direct the water in a downward flow, I usually start with my feet, just to get used to the temperature (rather like when you paddle in the sea), and then let the water flow down the thigh, knee, ankle and foot of first one and then the other leg. Then I take the showerhead up to one shoulder and let the water flow from each shoulder down each arm, and then down each side of the body (under the arms, flowing down to the hips).

After that I take a big breath and hold the showerhead over my head, letting the water flow from the crown, down the back of my head, neck and shoulders; then down the center of my back to my coccyx and buttocks; then from the crown down my face, throat and shoulders; then down the center of the front of my body over the heart, solar plexus, sacral and base chakras; and finishing by taking the water down the legs to the feet again. As I have already said, as soon as you have finished your cold shower you can turn the water up to warm or hot, however you like it, but the whole process will leave you feeling wonderfully clean, refreshed and invigorated.

If you don't have a shower at home, it is possible to buy shower attachments that will fit onto most bath taps, or you can use a jug instead. Just fill the washbasin with cold water, stand in the bath, and use the jug to pour the cold water over your chakras. Afterward, you can fill the washbasin (or your bath) with comfortably hot water and use it to warm yourself up, although a vigorous toweling or wrapping yourself in a terry-cloth robe will do the job too.

For most people, I recommend at least two cold showers a day:

1. First thing in the morning, to wash off any negative energies generated during the night, either from your own subconscious in dreams, or from the energy field of anyone you share your room with, as well as any possible energetic contamination picked up when returning from astral projection (there are theories that at least a part of our spirit rises out of our body when we sleep).

2. Then another one before bed, to wash off the negative "stuff" you pick up during an average day—including the energetic residue of any arguments or disagreements, negative comments and thoughts from people you have met, and even the misery and violence you may have seen on a television news program.

However, if you work in any of the caring professions, or as a therapist or counselor, or do any other work where you are frequently dealing with negative people, I would really recommend a cold shower as soon as you get in from work; it will get rid of any "psychic pollution" you have picked up during the day, and help you to feel refreshed and ready to enjoy your evening. You might also wish to change into clean casual clothes at this stage, to make you feel really fresh, but if not then just give your clothes a good shake before you put them back on, and if you have Second Degree, draw a Power Symbol over them, silently repeating its mantra three times and *intending* that the Reiki cleanse any negative energy from the clothing.

Using Reiki in Your Usual Cleansing Routine

In addition to using cold showers, you can enhance the effects of your usual cleansing routine with Reiki. When holding the showerhead in your hand, you can *intend* that Reiki flows out of your hand into the water, to cleanse and heal you as you shower; or if you have Second Degree, you can draw a Power Symbol over your showerhead before you begin. You can also draw the Power Symbol over your bath water, before you step into the bath (or when you are sitting in it if you happen to forget). If you don't know the symbols, simply *intend* that Reiki flows from your hands into your bath water, so that you are bathing in cleansing, healing water. Add a few drops of lavender oil, light some candles and you have the perfect remedial, relaxing retreat. (But do remember not to leave a burning candle unattended.)

Using Visualization for Cleansing

Another method of energetic cleansing involves using your thought energy in a visualization. It isn't as effective as a cold shower (sorry, there's no getting away from that!), but it helps when a real shower isn't available, and it is also a gentle and relaxing thing to do. Here's a visualization for you to try. You may find it useful to record it on tape, speaking slowly and rhythmically, in as relaxing a way as possible.

1. First, make yourself comfortable, either sitting or lying down, somewhere you can remain undisturbed for at least twenty minutes. Spend a few minutes tensing each group of muscles in turn, then letting them relax, from your toes right up to your facial muscles. When you are fully relaxed, you are ready to go on to the next stage.

2. Close your eyes and concentrate on your breathing. Let your breathing become slower and deeper, and begin to count your in-breaths: 1 and 2 and 3—let your breath come in as deeply as possible; 4 and 5 and 6—make sure you are expelling every bit of air on each out-breath; 7 and 8 and 9—your breathing is really deep and slow now; and 10... let your breath out with an audible sigh, but continue breathing in this slow, deep way.

3. Now imagine that you are standing on a path at the edge of a beautiful wood, and connect with all of your senses to bring this scene to life. You can feel the warmth of the sun on your skin, and feel a gentle breeze ruffling your hair. You can hear the leaves on nearby trees rustling in the breeze, and the songs of birds, too. Looking around you, you can see a beautiful blue sky, and the green of the grass, and the bright colors of flowers and butterflies. You can smell the sweet grass, and the breeze smells of pine and other woodland fragrances from the trees ahead. You can even imagine putting out your hand to touch a nearby leaf, or the bark of a tree.

4. Begin to walk along the path into the wood, where the sun is streaming down through the trees. As you walk, you hear the sound of running water, and the path seems to be leading you closer and closer to the sound.

5. Suddenly you come out of the trees into a sunlit glade, and at the far side of the glade is a beautiful waterfall, where the water runs into a deep blue pool that is surrounded by colorful flowers and long grasses. You walk toward the waterfall, and you feel the need to wash yourself clean in its sparkling water.

6. Quickly remove your clothing and step into the cool, sparkling water, letting it wash over your head and face and neck, over your shoulders and arms and hands, over the front and back of your body and legs, feeling it cleansing you and refreshing you.

7. When you feel really clean, you notice that the ribbons of water in the waterfall turn into ribbons of rainbow color, and your body is washed with red, orange and yellow light, and then with green and blue and indigo and violet light. As the rainbow colors fade away, you walk out of the waterfall, and take a dip in the beautiful blue pool.

8. The water of the pool is warm and relaxing, and it makes you feel playful, so you splash around for a few moments, enjoying the feel of the warm softness of the water.

9. As you climb out of the pool, you find a pile of lovely fresh, clean, white clothes waiting for you, which you put on. You turn toward the waterfall and the pool again, and acknowledge with thanks that you have been cleansed and purified. With a little bow of gratitude, you turn and walk back along the path, toward the entrance to the wood where you first started.

10. When you reach the edge of the wood, you spend a few moments just experiencing again the warmth of the sun, the scent of pine and fresh grass, the sight of the blue sky, enjoying it for a few moments longer.

11. Then the images begin to fade. Slowly, your awareness begins to return, and you can sense again the chair or bed beneath you,

and any sounds in the room. As your awareness returns fully, you can open your eyes. You will be back in the room where you first began this visualization, feeling peaceful, cleansed and refreshed.

TECHNIQUES FOR CLEANSING YOUR ENVIRONMENT

Where do you need to cleanse? Because you can potentially pick up negative energies anywhere, the answer should probably be "everywhere," but obviously that isn't practical! Basically, you need to regularly clean and cleanse all the areas in which you spend any substantial amount of time, and for most people that means their home and their workplace, or at least, their immediate surroundings at their place of work.

At home, the areas you need to concentrate on are the corners of each room, where negative or stagnant energy can collect, and places where you sit often, and especially where you sleep, so your bed and favorite chair are important. In the rest of this section I give a number of ideas on how to cleanse your environment; you can try them all and find out which ones you prefer.

You can also minimize the amount of negative energy that is brought into your home. One of the easiest ways of doing this is to remove your shoes (and ask guests to remove theirs) and leave them by the front (or back) door. This isn't just a method of avoiding dust or dirt soiling your carpets (although that is an added benefit)—it is a good technique for losing negative energy because this tends to be dense and "heavy," so that it is generally thickest at ground level. This means that in areas where there are lots of people, especially paved ones such as city streets, shopping centers, supermarkets, and so on, which have the greatest potential for being negative because of the numbers of people who use them, there is a layer of "sticky" negative energy lying around at ground level. Therefore when you walk in such areas, you are virtually wading through a "soup" of negative energy that will attach itself to your shoes; if you take them off by the door of your home, you will be limiting the effect of such negativity in your home.

One helpful way of getting rid of some of that negativity is to walk on a patch of natural earth—an area of grass is ideal—before you actually go back into your home, *intending* that any negativity leak back into the earth where it can be transformed and used. You can also stamp your feet vigorously a few times on a patch of grass, and this will help to shake loose much of the negative energy. It is also a particularly good idea not to have outdoor shoes in your bedroom, as you can be more susceptible to negative energies when you are asleep than when you are awake. An even better idea is to take off your shoes when you get home, walk barefoot or in slippers straight to your bathroom and have a cold shower, thereby getting rid of all the rest of the negativity you've picked up during the day.

Feng Shui and Principles of Clutter Clearing

Literally, the words feng shui mean "Wind-Water," but they are generally understood to represent the environment or "feel" of a place. The purpose of using feng shui is to help the occupants of any building (or room) to achieve success and prosperity, whatever that building or room is being used for—living, working, manufacturing, banking, and so on. However, feng shui can be applied to any space, so you can use the principles to create a calm, relaxing atmosphere in your home and any workspace you occupy.

The first and probably most important principle is to *clear the clutter* and always keep everything clean and tidy, so ensure that you clear your entire home (including the basement and attic) of all non-essential items. The idea is to get rid of everything you don't use or don't love, not to just stack things neatly or store them somewhere else. Tidying up is good, but it doesn't really tackle the main issue, which is that stuff you don't really love or no longer use just holds old energy, and it is this old energy that you need to clear out, just as much as the objects themselves. Doing a thorough clear-out can be quite a challenge, but the benefits really do outweigh the effort: you will probably find, as I did, that the energies feel so different that when your friends arrive in your newly cleared home they'll think it has been redecorated, or that you've done something special with the décor!

The Feng Shui Bagua

In feng shui any space is divided into an eight-sided figure called a bagua, and each part represents different aspects of your life. If you draw a plan of your home, or an individual room, the shape of the bagua can be superimposed on it so that you can see what areas of your life could be influenced by negative or positive energies. In general terms, energy flows around, through, over and under each space, entering and leaving buildings and rooms through doors and windows. It is believed that the most harmonious energies are created when a house has mountains behind it and a river in front, and faces due south—which means that few of us can live in ideal conditions!

To enhance the harmonic energies and create positivity and balance wherever you live or work, feng shui theories recommend various other things that are known as *cures*. Note that you musn't put any of these in place until after you have done a really good *spring-cleaning* and cleared all your clutter, otherwise you will simply enhance any negative energy, instead of attracting positive energy. Here are a few examples of feng shui "cures."

- ◆ **Mirrors** and **Lights** can reflect energy and create more positive space where parts of the bagua are missing (for example, in an oddly shaped room).

- ◆ **Wind Chimes** and **Mobiles** help to recirculate energy.

- ◆ **Plants** (healthy ones!) create growth.

- ◆ **Water** creates balance and/or flow.

- ◆ **Appropriate Artwork** can "lift" energies (or pull them down—it depends on the picture!).

- ◆ **Solid** and **Heavy Objects** can stop energies flowing through too quickly.

◆ **Colors** can create an atmosphere, so decorating your home in harmonious colors to provide a well-balanced feel is helpful. Soft colors are best: pale green, blue, pink or lilac are the most restful—but white is also good.

Although the bagua is usually drawn as an octagonal figure, when using it in rooms or a whole building it is often easier to draw it as a series of nine squares (*see below*). The ideal then is to place furniture or objects in appropriate places. A brief description of what each area represents is given on the following pages. The bagua doesn't have to

4	9	2
Fortunate Blessings Wealth, Abundance	Illumination Fame, Self-expression, Achievement of Enlightenment	Relationships Marriage, Intimacy
3	5	7
Elders Family, Ancestors, Heritage	Unity T'ai Chi, Health	Creativity Offspring, Children, Projects
8	1	6
Contemplation Inner Knowledge, Self-realisation	The Journey Career, Path in Life	Helpful People Friends, Angels, Guides

This bottom line should be aligned with the wall
that has the door leading into the home or room.

be square—it can be oblong with the shortest sides at the top and bottom, or with the shortest sides to the left and right.

Draw a plan of the shape of your room (or home), then divide it up into nine equal squares to see which part is which. The bottom line of the diagram is the one that represents the wall where the entrance door is to the home or the room. If your room or home has an odd shape—perhaps it has a bay window, or is L-shaped—the bagua will still cover the areas of the room or house that are "missing." For example, an L-shaped room or apartment might have no area of Relationships, or the area of Fortunate Blessings might be missing. Place a mirror on a wall so that the reflection in the mirror "projects" into the missing space—but make sure that what it reflects is pleasant, like a plant or a beautiful picture, otherwise the "cure" won't make much difference!

1. **The Journey** This area is to do with your working life, how you earn money, your general approach and your spiritual path through life, and it is also an area of new beginnings and opportunities.

2. **Relationships** This obviously concerns your intimate relationship with partners, but is also about how you relate to yourself, and to other people in general—friends, family, colleagues.

3. **Elders** This is the area that relates to your heritage, ancestors, parents, authority figures and influences from the past—perhaps it's a good place to have a photograph of Dr. Usui and your Reiki Master(s)?

4. **Fortunate Blessings** This is about the flow of universal abundance into your life, so it is not just about money or material possessions, but includes all types of prosperity, blessings and anything good that you attract into your life.

5. **Unity (also known as T'ai Chi)** This is the area governing health and general energy levels, so it's a particularly important place to keep clean and clear!

6. **Helpful People** This area is about help from family, friends, colleagues, authority figures, people you've never met and even sources of information such as books. It includes help from unseen guides, angels and earth spirits, so it's a good place to keep a picture of angels, fairies, and so on.

7. **Creativity** Although this is traditionally seen as the area of off-spring or children, it also covers anything else that you create or give birth to in the world, so it includes manifesting more good things in your life, as well as art, poetry and music.

8. **Contemplation** This area is associated with learning, study, introspection, meditation, intuition, inner guidance and your Higher Self, or anything that enhances your spiritual focus, so perhaps a meditation stool, a small altar and some inspirational books on a shelf would be a good idea here.

9. **Illumination** This area refers to your individuality and uniqueness, how you express yourself in the world, what "lights up your life," your reputation or what you are renowned or "famous" for. On a higher level it is about inspiration, spiritual enlightenment and self-actualization, so this could be another good area to use for meditation.

Using Reiki for Clearing, Cleansing and Creating Sacred Space

You can use Reiki to clear, harmonize and protect any spaces you occupy, and the most effective way of doing this is to place Power Symbols in each corner of each room, on the floor and ceiling and also on any furniture where you spend lots of time, such as your bed or favorite chair, and imagine and *intend* that the whole room be filled with Reiki. Even if you don't have Second Degree, you can still use Reiki for cleansing. Just sit quietly and visualize and *intend* that Reiki flows from your palms to fill the whole room with healing energy and light, perhaps imagining the light of Reiki flowing like a soft mist until it fills the whole space.

Using Sounds and Scents for Cleansing

Certain sound vibrations can have a cleansing effect, and a good way to use sound to cleanse rooms is to make "noise" in the corners in order to break up stagnant energy. This can be as simple as clapping your hands together firmly a few times, or you can bang on a drum, or use a Tibetan bell or singing bowl, for example. Your own voice can also be used, and "toning" an om is a good way to do this.

Scents are also vibrational, and you can use aromatherapy oils or incense sticks to help with cleansing. I find that a few drops each of lemon oil and lavender oil in water in an oil burner are best for cleansing spaces, and the smell is both pleasant and refreshing. One or two lit incense sticks, wafted into the corners of a room, also provide a nice way of cleansing a space. If you have Second Degree you can combine this method with drawing out the shape of the Power Symbol, *intending* that Reiki lightens and clears an area of all negative energies: this is an excellent cleansing technique.

The Ceremonial Use of Smudge

Another way of employing a combination of scent and smoke for cleansing involves using a smudge stick or smudge mix. "Smudge" is the name given to a combination of herbs that the Native Americans use for cleansing physically and spiritually. The herbs most commonly used are sage (usually *Salvia apiana*, white sage), cedar (western red cedar, *Thuja plicata* or Californian incense cedar, *Calocedrus descurrens*) and sweetgrass (*Hierochloe odorata*). Sage is used to banish negative energies, cleanse and purify; cedar is used to balance male/female energies; and sweetgrass is said to bring sweetness, beauty and forgiveness into one's life and surroundings. Occasionally, other herbs, such as lavender (*Lavandula officinalis*), are included in the mix to bring spiritual blessings.

The dried herbs can either be in a wand, where long strands of the herbs are tied into a bundle, or are available as a dried mix of seeds, leaves and small pieces. Sweetgrass is usually braided into a long plait, tied at each end. The ceremonial use of smudge involves setting light to the herbs so that they smolder and produce a cleansing smoke, which is then wafted around the area that needs cleansing, or around and through a person's auric field. The wands are the easiest to deal with, as they catch light fairly quickly and smolder for several minutes, which is usually enough time to waft the smoke into each corner and along each wall of a room.

To smudge someone, first get them to stand with their arms held out at the sides, level with their shoulders. Take a smoldering smudge wand and pass it over the top of their head and shoulders two or three times, taking care at all times not to get the wand too close to their hair, face or clothing. Then pass the smudge wand along the top and underneath each arm, and gracefully zigzag the smoke down the front of the face, body and legs, and then again at the back of the head and down the back of the body and the legs. Finally, ask the person to lift one foot at a time, and waft the smudge smoke under the sole of each foot. You may need to relight the smudge stick several times to keep it smoking.

To smudge yourself, the traditional way is to waft the smoke toward you using a large feather—preferably one that you have found specifically for that purpose. Hold the smoldering herb wand in one hand and the feather in the other, then "brush" the smoke toward you with the feather, from the top of your head down to your feet. Waft the smoke over your shoulders so that it flows down your back, taking care not to get the smoldering wand too close to your hair, skin or clothing. You can also do this under each arm.

I find this a very relaxing thing to do, and the smell is lovely, too. Many people can really notice the difference in their energy field after smudging—it feels light and clear, and this often has an energizing effect, so it's good to do it in the morning or if you're facing a difficult task of some kind. For safety reasons, do remember to put out the smudge when you've finished—putting it into a metal container like a saucepan with a lid is the easiest and safest way: it will go out quickly when it is starved of oxygen.

chapter 5

SELF-TREATMENT WITH REIKI

The first and most obvious place to start on your self-healing with Reiki is to carry out self-treatments. In this chapter I suggest a number of different ways of treating yourself with Reiki as the best and most comprehensive part of your essential maintenance program for physical, mental, emotional and spiritual health. Whichever type of self-treatment you use—the standard twelve hand positions, the "Whole Body, Whole Self" treatment, or the "Mental and Emotional" treatment—because the hand positions cover the whole of you, and because Reiki works holistically, a self-treatment helps all of you, body, mind, emotions and spirit, to reach a state of harmony and balance.

I strongly recommend that you give yourself a treatment every day, preferably one lasting at least half an hour, although longer is even better—and of course you don't have to limit yourself to only one treatment a day. Giving yourself Reiki is a loving act to yourself, as well as being a very comforting and relaxing thing to do, so the more treatments you have the better.

TIME AND PLACE

It is recommended that each hand position on the head and front and back of the body be held for between three and five minutes, and that hand positions on the arms and legs be held for between one and two minutes. How you do the timing is up to you, but because I prefer to close my eyes during a self-treatment I count the seconds in my head, which I also find to be a very meditative activity. Alternatively, listening to a ticking clock is useful for this, as there is usually one tick per second. Another possibility is to buy a CD or tape with gentle music that is played in definite three- or five-minute slots and has either silence or a soft gong sound between each section to let you know when to move your hands to a new position. Such CDs are available commercially, but it is easy enough to record your own. That way you can tailor them specifically to the amount of time you prefer, and use music that you particularly like.

However, the actual number of minutes isn't what is crucial; it's the fact that you are giving yourself Reiki that matters! You can just allow your hands to stay in each position for as long as you feel is needed, and use your intuition to let you know when to move on—the more practice you get in self-treatment, the easier it is to let the Reiki guide you.

Self-treatments can be carried out almost anywhere and at any time of day, but they are most comfortable if you are lying in bed or sitting in a comfortable chair, so that your body and arms are well supported. I prefer to do mine first thing in the morning, almost as soon as I wake up, although I do set my alarm clock to ring again about forty minutes later in case I get so relaxed that I drift back to sleep. It is also really pleasant to do a self-treatment last thing at night, although if you are tired you probably won't get very far before drifting off into peaceful sleep.

Don't feel you have to force yourself to keep to a particular time. Any time that is convenient to you, that fits in with your lifestyle, is the best time, because that way you'll feel more relaxed so you'll enjoy the experience more. The benefits of giving yourself daily self-treatments are cumulative—the more Reiki you receive, the better Reiki is able to remove blockages and promote deep healing on all levels.

SENSATIONS IN YOUR HANDS AND BODY

One thing you need to bear in mind is that when you are treating yourself you rarely get as much sensation in your hands as when you are treating other people. I have been self-treating for over twenty years, and unless I'm treating areas of my body that are sore, aching or injured, I rarely feel anything at all in my hands, and most of my students report the same thing. Don't worry if this happens to you, as it doesn't mean the Reiki isn't flowing; you will probably get other indications, anyway, such as feeling very relaxed or sleepy.

The most likely reason for getting little sensation when treating yourself is that, as I have explained earlier in this book, Reiki is really your own Soul energy, so of course it is resonating in harmony with your own life force already, because your life force is vibrating in similar wave patterns, albeit at a lower vibrationary level. When you treat other people your energies are vibrating quite differently, and this is why you are more aware of feelings in your hands.

If, however, you do experience quite a lot of sensation in your hands, such as heat, cold, tingles or other vibrations when treating specific areas, or if you feel those sensations in the part of your body you are treating, do continue to let the Reiki flow there, as this is usually an indication that more healing is needed. Just leave your hands in place until the sensation lessens—you don't need to time the hand positions to the exact second. The timings are a rough guide, and there is no reason why you cannot have your hands in the same position for half an hour or more if you feel you need to.

DETECTING ENERGETIC IMBALANCES BEFORE SELF-TREATMENT

Byosen Reikan-ho

It is possible to sense energetic imbalances with your hands before you carry out a self-treatment by scanning your body. In the Japanese tradition this technique is called *Byosen Reikan-ho*: *Byo* means "sickness, disease or imbalance"; *Sen* means "before, ahead, previous, future"; *Rei* means "spirit or soul"; *Kan* means "feeling, sensation or emotion"; and *Ho* means "treatment, method or way."

Because illness or disease is present as a dense or sticky energy patch in the energy field before it manifests as a physical condition, this

79

technique is excellent for warding off physical problems by detecting them first in the aura, allowing you to treat them with Reiki before they reach the physical level. The type and amount of sensation that can be detected in the hands will vary from person to person, depending upon the severity and condition of any imbalance or "dis-ease" (physical or energetic), and can include tingling, tickling, pulsating, piercing, stinging, pain, numbness, heat, cold, and so on. In Japanese these sensations are called *Hibiki*, and they normally oc-cur only in the hands, but can occasionally be felt in the arms or even up to the shoulders in extreme cases.

1. Start by sitting or standing comfortably.

2. Spend a few moments centering yourself with your hands in the *Gassho* position, and allow your mind to become calm. Then *intend* to activate your intuitive ability to detect energetic imbal-ances—you could say silently to yourself "I begin *Byosen Reikan-ho* now" or "I begin using Reiki to sense and heal energetic imbalances now."

3. Place one or both your hands, palms downward, slightly (five to fifteen centimeters/two to six inches) above your body starting at your head, over the crown chakra, and begin to move them slowly down your body. Sometimes it is helpful to close your eyes, so that you can "tune in" more easily to any sensations in your hands. You will probably find that there is a general "background" sensation of gentle warmth or tingling or even a cool breeze when you pass your hands over one of your major chakras. However, some areas will feel different, and these are the areas of *Byosen*. The more you practice, the easier it will become to identify the subtle differences, but pay attention to changes in heat or tingling, or any of the other sensations detailed above.

4. When you sense a difference in the energy field, hold your hands on or over that area. The sensations will ebb and flow in natural cycles, increasing and then decreasing. Don't automatically assume that when the sensation reduces it is time to move your hands, as

these cycles will continue for as long as your hands are on your body. The longer you hold your hands over a particular place the more energy cycles you will feel, but with each cycle the intensity will diminish, so keep your hands in place for at least one cycle, and if you have time keep your hands in the same place until there is virtually no discernible difference in sensation (that is, until there is more of a continuous sensation than an ebb and flow).

5. When you are ready, move your hands gently and slowly to the next area of *Byosen* and repeat step 4.

6. When you have completed *Byosen Reikan-ho* over your whole body, place your hands at midchest height in the *Gassho* position, and silently give thanks for the Reiki, bowing slightly as a mark of respect.

SELF-TREATMENT HAND POSITIONS

When you attended your first Reiki course you were probably taught a series of twelve hand positions for a full self-treatment, following the chakras down the body starting with four on the head and then four down the front of the body, and another four down the back, although there might be slight variations in the exact positioning of the hands, depending upon which Master you trained with. Each hand position should be easy to do, and feel comfortable, otherwise you won't get the full benefit in terms of relaxation. Your hands should be laid gently on your body in the order shown below, and it is usual to keep your fingers close together, with the thumbs also close to your forefingers.

Each hand is placed on its corresponding side of the body, partly because this is comfortable, but also because treating each side of the body equally helps to balance the energies, encouraging a good flow of Ki around the body's energy system so that it is more effective. However, using only one hand is not detrimental in any way if you have any form of disability or injury that prevents you from using two hands, such as a broken arm, a stroke or an amputation. Simply place one hand on one side, and *intend*, or visualize, that the other hand is in a complementary position on the other side. Energy follows intentional thought, so the Reiki will flow through appropriate parts of your energy body—even if an arm or leg is amputated, its subtle energy counterparts are still there—and then into wherever you intend it to go.

It is traditional to begin the treatment at the head, and the first few hand positions focus the Reiki particularly on the crown and third-eye chakras. The hand position on the neck works on the throat chakra, the next position on the heart chakra, and so on, until the whole body and all the major chakras have been treated. Energy can easily flow into and out of the body through any of the chakras, but when it flows into the crown chakra first this seems to accelerate the effect, allowing the Reiki to flow even more easily into the other chakras, and it also promotes a particularly gentle, calming and relaxing effect.

If the energy is taken in first through the base chakra or the feet, it is in no way harmful, but it tends to have a more vibrant and energizing effect, which some people can find slightly agitating. However, please feel free to experiment. You might like it! Hard-and-fast rules aren't really compatible with the ethos of Reiki, so although I suggest certain ways of using it that are good basic foundation techniques, after some practice do let Reiki guide you to use it in ways that feel good for you.

INTENTION AND INVOCATION

Reiki doesn't need any complicated rituals before it will start to flow. All it takes is your *intention* to use Reiki, which can if you wish be accompanied by a simple invocation such as "Let Reiki flow into me now for my highest and greatest good." Thoughts are a form of energy and can be very powerful, especially if they have the force of intention behind them, but Reiki will actually begin to flow from the moment you first think of using it, so as you place your hands on your body to begin self-healing, it is already flowing.

Note that where and how Reiki flows is not up to you—you are merely a channel for this healing energy. Because it is divinely guided it goes where it is needed, not necessarily where you decide you would like it to go. Having the *intention* that it should flow for the highest and greatest good therefore helps to get rid of the ego that might otherwise be involved.

You may, for example, really want to heal a particular illness, or to get rid of some physical symptoms, but it might be for your greatest and highest good for these symptoms to remain until you are ready to face up to the causative issues, so Reiki will go first to the causative levels—mental, emotional or spiritual. It may also bring some temporary relief of symptoms, but you can never guarantee what Reiki will do because it is never under your conscious control, even when you are treating yourself. Sadly, this means that you need to get rid of any specific expectations as to the outcome of self-treatment. This can be very hard, I know, because it is human nature to want to feel physically well. But do realize that by channeling Reiki into yourself you are helping yourself, even if that help doesn't turn out to be exactly what you had hoped it would be.

PREPARING FOR A SELF-TREATMENT

Whatever time of day you do your self-treatment you will presumably already have decided where you are going to carry it out—sitting in a comfortable chair or cross-legged on the floor, lying on a bed or maybe even on a lounge chair on the beach. Before you start, however, it is a good idea to do one of the self-cleansing techniques, such as *Kenyoku-ho* (*see pages 59–61*) or the Reiki shower (*see pages 56–58*), and then spend a few moments just gently breathing deeply and evenly to center yourself, and allowing your body to relax. You might even choose to do a full *Hatsurei-ho* (*see pages 58–64*) before your self-treatment, which can make it a particularly relaxing and effective way to start or end the day. I personally prefer to close my eyes during a self-treatment, and then, as I raise my hands to place them in the first position, I think and *intend* that I am beginning a self-treatment, and think and *intend* that the Reiki will flow into me for my highest and greatest good.

THE TRADITIONAL SELF-TREATMENT

As I have mentioned above, the traditional self-treatment usually consists of twelve hand positions: four on the head, four on the front of the body and four on the back. As all of these positions form part of the more extensive "Whole Body, Whole Self" treatment, you will find all of them described fully in the next section. To help you identify them, here are the reference numbers from that treatment next to the numbered positions for the traditional self-treatment.

Traditional Self-treatment	**"Whole Body, Whole Self"**
Hand Positions	Hand Positions
1. Over the eyes	No. 2
2. Then the ears	No. 3
3. The back of the head	No. 4
4. The neck	No. 5
5. The chest	No. 6
6. The solar plexus	No. 7
7. The navel	No. 8
8. The pelvic area	No. 9
9. The shoulders	No. 10
10. The back (midway between neck and waist)	No. 15
11. The back of the waist	No. 16
12. The buttocks	No. 17

This is of course an excellent way of treating yourself with Reiki. Traditionally you maintain each hand position for between three and five minutes, so that the treatment lasts between half an hour and an hour. This allows Reiki to flow around your whole body and into your aura. However, by extending the number of hand positions it is possible to have an even more comprehensive treatment, so I am going to suggest a slightly different approach that I call a "Whole Body, Whole Self" treatment to distinguish it from the traditional self-treatment above.

"WHOLE BODY, WHOLE SELF" TREATMENT

The traditional self-treatment does treat the whole body, as I have already said, but it has its limitations, because there are parts of the body that don't directly receive treatment—the arms, hands, legs and feet. While sometimes people are taught to include these limbs when treating themselves or others, these hand positions are frequently left out—although of course your arms and legs do receive some Reiki, because it will flow through the body's energy meridians to those areas, especially when you treat the shoulders, chest, pelvic area and buttocks.

On a metaphysical level, the arms and legs are pretty important, as they are the "moving centers" and the means by which we interact physically and directly with life. They represent movement and flexibility, expression and creativity, and reveal whether we embrace life fully or hold back, how we "hold on" and "get a grip on things," how we move forward in life, whether we step out confidently, or "put our foot in it," among other things. So treating them with Reiki directly can have lots of beneficial effects, such as allowing the stored emotions they hold to be released, as you will see later.

I also suggest starting the treatment with your hands over the crown, which is an additional hand position designed to open up your energy field quickly so that it is especially receptive to the Reiki. It immediately sends the Reiki from the crown down the Hara line, the energy line that connects all of the major chakras, thereby activating all of your energy centers. This might not be a familiar starting point for you, but I would really recommend that you give this new format a try—I think you will find it a very useful and effective method of self-treatment. Perhaps you could do the more familiar twelve-hand-position treatment on weekdays, and the longer twenty-two-position "Whole Body, Whole Self" treatment during the weekends, when you have more time, if that fits in with your life pattern.

I have suggested timings for each hand position, but of course you can use your intuition to decide to treat any area for a shorter time, or for longer if you sense that it needs it. I have also provided a general guide to what *might* be treated by each hand position, on both a physical and a metaphysical basis, although of course every hand position is in effect treating the whole of the body, because Reiki flows into and around the whole subtle energy and physical bodies through the meridians. It also affects the mental, emotional and spiritual aspects of the person, healing or "wholing" and bringing everything into harmony and balance. Remember that Reiki will always go where it is needed most, without requiring any conscious control from you, so it will always work for your greatest and highest good.

The Hand Positions

The twenty-two hand positions for the "Whole Body, Whole Self" treatment are given in four sections:

1. The head and front of the body.

2. The shoulders, arms and hands.

3. The back of the body.

4. The legs and feet.

I find it best to do them in this order, as it seems fairly logical to me, but again, feel free to experiment. You might do the head and front of the body (positions 1–9), followed immediately by the back of the body (positions 10 and 15–17), and then finish off with the arms and legs. Just see how it feels for you, and "go with the flow." Of course, the additional ten hand positions will take extra time, and I suggest that you generally keep your hands in place for between one and two minutes each for the arms, hands, legs and feet. You may, however, initially feel drawn to spending three to five minutes on these hand positions, the same as for the rest of the body. This is because if you haven't been treating them regularly before you will probably find, as I did, that your hands get pretty hot as the Reiki flows in and helps to release areas of blockage that haven't been activated much before. As always, the more time you can give yourself for self-treatment the better.

The Head and Front of the Body

The nine hand positions covering the head and the front of the body work to activate and balance all of the seven major chakras, and treat all of the major organs and systems of the body, so they are the perfect start to your self-treatment. The first four hand positions, on the crown, over the eyes, over the ears and over the back of the head, work together: they cover the head and the whole of the brain with all of its functions and control mechanisms for the whole body, from memory to movement, including the nervous system and the endocrine system.

1. THE CROWN

Physically, this hand position allows Reiki to flow into the crown chakra and the whole of the head and brain, the nervous system and the endocrine system—especially the pineal and pituitary glands, which are both located in the brain. Metaphysically, Reiki flowing from this hand position particularly encourages inner knowledge and awareness, spirituality, a sense of unity and connectedness to everyone and everything, and feelings of fulfillment, completion and enlightenment.

Place both hands, one hand crossed over the other, on the crown of your head. *Intend* that Reiki should flow to open up your energy field

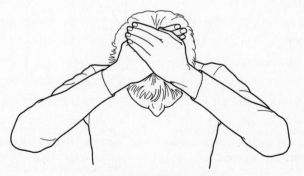

Hand position for the crown.

so that it becomes even more receptive to its healing energies, and keep your hands in that position for between three and five minutes.

2. THE EYES

In this position, Reiki flows into both the crown and brow chakras, and once again into the whole head and brain, nervous system and endocrine system, including the pituitary and pineal glands, as well as specifically into the eyes and face. On a metaphysical level, Reiki flowing here can encourage intuition, insight and imagination, sometimes promoting the development of inner vision, clairvoyance or other psychic gifts.

3. THE EARS

Reiki again flows into the crown and brow chakras, but here it is also connected with the throat chakra. It treats the head, brain, nervous system, and endocrine system including the pituitary and pineal glands, as well as the ears, sinuses, nose and face. Other benefits of Reiki flowing here include not only the physical ability to hear, but also the willingness to listen to higher guidance, and the possible development of clairaudiant skills. This position also works to promote healthy sleep patterns.

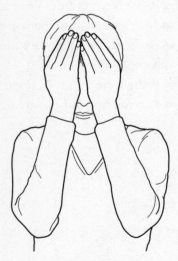 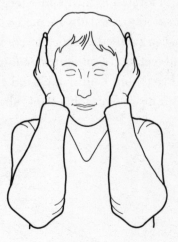

One hand held loosely over each eye, with the heel of each hand placed on your cheekbones, fingertips on your brow. (Three to five minutes.)

One hand held loosely cupped over each ear, with the heel of each hand placed level with the earlobe, and the fingertips pointing upward toward the temples. (Three to five minutes.)

4. THE BACK OF THE HEAD

Reiki flowing into the back of the head will, as before, cover the crown and brow chakras, and the brain, nervous system and endocrine system, including the pituitary and pineal glands, but because it also flows into the visual cortex, it can help both with physical sight and inner vision, often activating the imagination and stimulating visualization. However, it also helps to promote restful sleep. Whichever of the following alternative hand positions you use, hold it for three to five minutes.

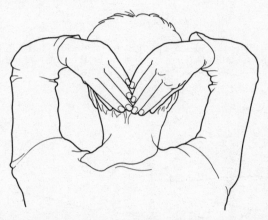

4a. Both hands next to each other at the back of the head, pointing downward with the fingertips at the base of the skull.

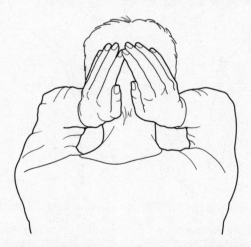

4b. As an alternative, you can place your hands next to each other at the back of the head, with the heel of each hand level with the base of the skull, fingertips pointing toward the crown.

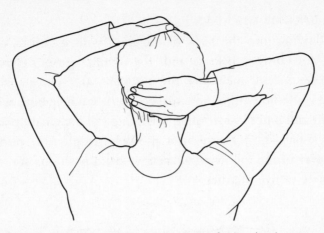

4c. My favorite alternative, which is particularly comforting, but is not normally a part of the traditional hand positions, is one hand on the crown of the head, and the other covering the back of the head.

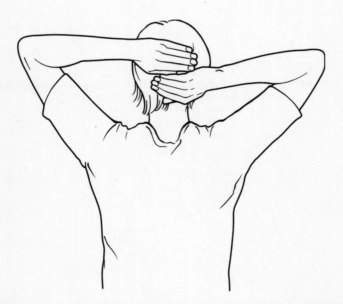

4d. Another very comforting hand position is to place one hand cradling the base of the skull, with the other just above it.

5. THE THROAT

This hand position allows Reiki to flow into the throat chakra, and on a physical level it flows into the neck, throat, tonsils, adenoids and vocal cords, as well as into the jaw, mouth, teeth, gums, nose, sinuses and ears. It also flows into the thyroid and parathyroid glands, which control metabolism and growth. On a metaphysical level, Reiki flowing from this hand position encourages the ability to communicate honestly and effectively, and promotes creativity and self-expression, including expression through music and the voice. Whichever of the alternative hand positions you use, hold it for three to five minutes.

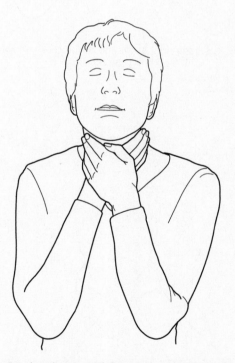

5a. One hand on top of the other, covering the throat.

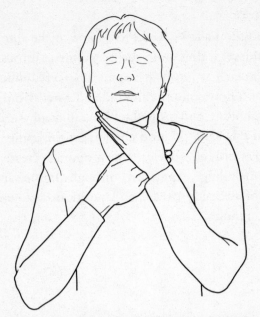

5b. Alternatively, one hand right at the top of the chest, and the other hand covering the throat.

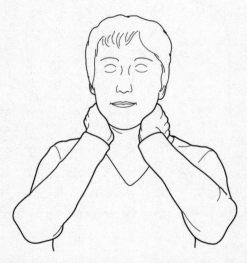

5c. Another alternative is to have one hand on each side of the neck, and it is OK to have the heels of the hands touching, or slightly apart.

6. THE CHEST

Reiki in this hand position flows into the heart chakra, and physically it has a particularly wide influence, as it works on the heart and the entire cardiovascular system, the lymphatic system, the immune system, the lungs and the whole of the respiratory system, and the thymus gland, as well as the arms and hands. Metaphysically, Reiki flowing here encourages unconditional love and good relationships, empathy, kindness and compassion toward others and oneself, self-acceptance and understanding, and a willingness to both give and receive. Whichever of the following hand positions you use, hold it for three to five minutes.

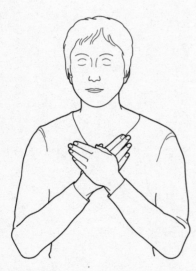
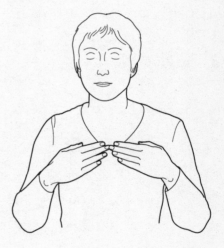

6a. Both hands crossed in the center of the chest, over the heart chakra.

6b. Or alternatively, one hand on each side of the chest, very slightly above each breast. The fingertips can touch in the center, or be slightly apart.

7. THE SOLAR PLEXUS

Here Reiki flows into the solar plexus chakra, and this is another place where Reiki can help a wide variety of physical and metaphysical conditions. From here Reiki flows into the liver, spleen, pancreas, gallbladder, stomach and the whole of the digestive system. It will help you to develop willpower, self-control, a recognition of your need for personal authority and autonomy, self-esteem and self-determination, as well as an understanding of your potential and your purpose in life. Additionally, it encourages an increase in your overall energy.

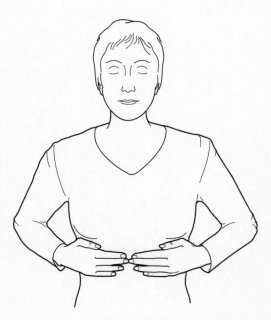

One hand on each side of the body, covering the solar plexus (midriff). Again, the fingertips can touch in the center, or be slightly apart. (Three to five minutes.)

8. THE WAIST/NAVEL

From this position Reiki flows into the sacral chakra, and physically into another wide range of organs and conditions, including the kidneys and adrenal glands (adrenal cortex and adrenal medulla), the lower digestive organs, the prostate, bladder and entire urinary tract and the female reproductive system—the uterus and ovaries. It therefore has an effect on an individual's sexuality, emotions and romantic relationships, aspects of intimacy and sharing, and all facets of sensuality, including the appetite for food, sex and other pleasures. In addition, it encourages creativity in all its forms, and an appreciation of all the senses.

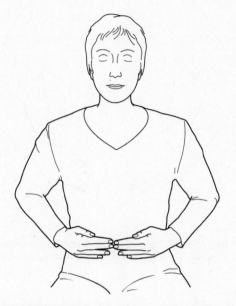

One hand on each side of the body, fingers pointing toward each other, at about the same level as your navel, which can be either very slightly above or below your natural waistline. (Three to five minutes.)

9. THE PELVIC AREA

From this hand position, Reiki flows into the base or root chakra, and also into the body's structure, including the whole skeleton, the muscles, skin and blood, the bladder, the bowel and elimination system, the genitals and again into the reproductive organs, as well as the pelvis, hips, legs and feet. Metaphysically, Reiki flows here into your feelings about your physical body, as well as your feelings of security and trust and sense of survival; this covers issues about money, home, work, your sense of belonging and your interaction with nature and the Earth.

95

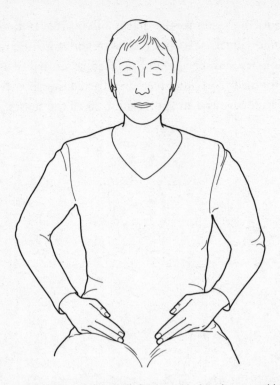

One hand on each side of the body, fingers pointing downward but slightly diagonally in a V shape, sloping toward the pelvic area. (Three to five minutes.)

The Shoulders, Arms and Hands

The shoulders and arms are centers of activity, enabling us to interact physically with people and things. They can indicate how much effort we put into life, how we express ourselves and how we embrace life itself. Do we enjoy cuddles, hugging people and holding them close, or do we prefer to "shrug them off" and hold them "at arm's length"? How do we "handle" life and all it problems? Do we "hold on" to things or people for too long, or let them "slip through our grasp"? Are we comfortable with close contact, with gentle stroking, caressing or tickling with humor and love, or do we need to keep a "firm grip" on life and the people close to us, or even prefer slapping with our hands or punching with our fists as a way of communicating what we feel?

Of course, our hands also enable us to carry out a huge range of tasks, from personal activities such as washing, dressing and cooking, to practical work like gardening, car maintenance or typing, and creative pursuits such as carving, embroidery or playing the piano, so any lack of physical dexterity can have a great impact on our lives as a whole.

10. THE SHOULDERS

In the traditional twelve-hand-position self-treatment, this position is the start of treating the back. However, when Reiki flows into this hand position it flows not only into the shoulders, but also down into the arms and hands, so I have included it in this section. Physically the shoulders are where most of us hold a lot of tension and stress, and this can cause general aches and pains, including headaches, so this hand position treats the muscles and joints in the shoulders, as well as the upper back. From a metaphysical perspective, the shoulders are where we carry responsibility, often "shouldering" other people's burdens, and where we hold on to the stress of not doing what we want to do, so Reiki flows into these feelings to encourage relaxation and a more realistic perspective. Whichever of the alternative hand positions you use, hold it for three to five minutes.

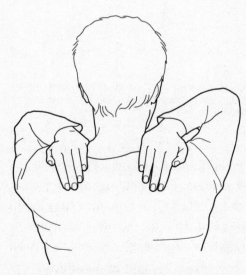 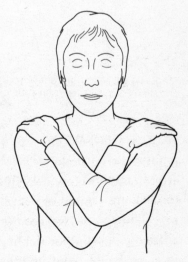

10a. Place one hand on top of each shoulder, or if you find this uncomfortable try 10b.

10b. Place one hand on top of each shoulder by crossing your arms in front of your chest.

11. THE UPPER ARMS

The arms represent our ability to embrace life and all its experiences, as well as to interact with people. The upper arms are usually quite strong, so as well as treating the arms physically, Reiki flowing into this hand position helps to let feelings and energy flow actively from the shoulder downward, to help us to take control of our lives, to let go of resistance to expressing our feelings, so that we can express courage and strength in a caring and gentle way—through a hug rather than a crushing embrace!

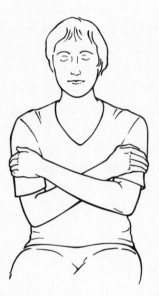

Crossing your arms in front of your chest, place your left hand on your right upper arm, and your right hand on your left upper arm. Hold this position for between one and two minutes.

12. THE ELBOWS

Joints need to move freely and flexibly, and the elbow joints enable our arms to respond to a wide range of needs, from holding someone close to wielding a spade in the garden, so Reiki can flow into the elbows to encourage freedom of movement. But the elbow can represent changing directions and accepting new experiences on a metaphysical level, so Reiki flows here to encourage strength and enthusiasm— what we call "elbow grease"—to come into our lives, and to give us the flexibility and the ability to adapt to different life situations.

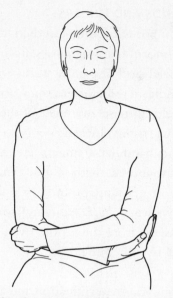

Place one hand on each elbow for one to two minutes.

13. THE FOREARMS

As in position 11, letting Reiki flow into the arms helps the heart energy, flowing down our arms, to express love and acceptance and encourage our ability to grasp hold of life in all its forms.

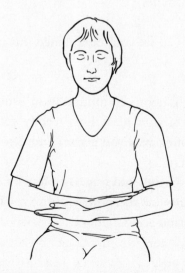

Place one hand on each forearm for one to two minutes.

99

14. THE WRISTS, HANDS AND FINGERS

The wrists are very important joints, and their wide range of movement enables us to perform many activities, from hitting a tennis ball to cradling a baby's head. Stiff or painful wrists will limit what we are able to do and may indicate resistance to some activity, so Reiki flowing into the wrists helps to raise awareness of the issue or activity we are avoiding and to free up the blocked energy so that we can take any necessary action. The hands and fingers are especially important, because we use them to interact with so much in our lives—touching or caressing, holding or grasping, pushing or pulling—so if they are stiff or painful it shows we are not "handling" some aspect of life too well, and are withdrawing from the action. Even problems with individual fingers can tell us something:

◆ The thumb is about your determination and about feeling in control of your own destiny.

◆ The index finger represents how you view yourself and your place in the world.

◆ The middle finger is about self-discipline, responsibility and the effort you put into life.

◆ The ring finger is about your confidence, imagination and instinctive feelings.

◆ The little finger is about communication issues such as how well you can put across your ideas, how readily you appreciate others' viewpoints and how well you get on with people generally.

Reiki flows into the hands and fingers to free up blocked energy and to raise awareness of what issues we need to look into to regain and maintain our dexterity.

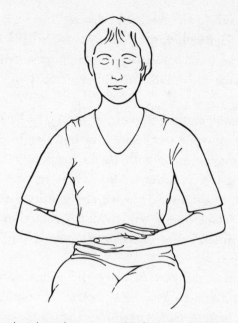

Place your hands so that the palms are roughly facing each other, with the fingertips
of each hand covering the opposite wrist. Hold this position for a minimum of two
minutes, although because you are treating three areas—the wrists, hands and
fingers—it will be beneficial to treat them for longer, say three to five minutes. (Also,
if you have particular problems with dexterity you can treat each position separately,
that is the wrist, then the hand and finally the fingers on each side.)

The Back of the Body

Although all the hand positions on the front of the body enable
Reiki to flow around the whole body, and therefore into the back as
well, treating the back separately allows Reiki to flow even more
effectively into some particular parts of the body. The spine, for
example, is a very important part of our skeleton, and the support
structure for our lives both physically and metaphysically. The four
hand positions on the back (that is, including the shoulders, *see page
97*) treat the whole of the spine from the base of the neck down to
the coccyx, as well as treating other vital areas again, such as the
lungs, liver and kidneys.

Millions of people have what are broadly termed "back problems,"
which may seem to have fairly obvious physical causes—poor

posture when sitting or standing, twisting into awkward positions, lifting heavy weights without due care, and so on, but at a metaphysical level the back is seen as your support system, and different areas of the back are linked to different areas of support in our everyday lives.

Issues of survival, earning a living or having to be the "backbone" of your family or your workplace can translate into fear, anger or guilt, so treating the back with Reiki helps to release and transmute these negative emotions. Also, when we are called upon to put an effort into things we say we are "putting our back into it," so if we're reluctant or resistant to doing something we may "put our back out" instead, as an alternative to saying "no" to someone or something!

You may find it difficult to place the palms of your hands flat against your body when treating your back if you have any stiffness in your wrists or fingers, for example if you have arthritis. If this is the case, just place the *backs* of your hands against your body instead. The palm chakra, like all the other chakras, spreads out from both sides, so Reiki will flow out of the back of your hand, and also out of your fingers, if that is what it needs to do. I describe the alternative positions below.

15. THE BACK

This hand position is roughly halfway between your shoulders and your waist, so it is treating primarily the upper portion of your back, your heart and your lungs, as well as your heart and solar plexus chakras. This section of the back is linked with feeling emotionally unsupported, unloved or misunderstood; the heart is naturally linked to love and joy, and the lungs are connected to deep-seated issues about our capacity for, or fear of, life itself. Whichever alternative hand position you adopt, hold it for between three and five minutes.

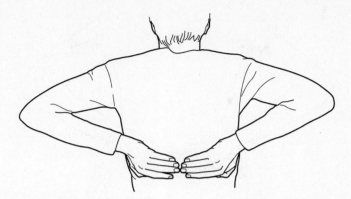

15a. Place both hands, palms flat, one on each side of your back, preferably positioned midway between your shoulders and waist, but if this is difficult, then as high above your waist as you can comfortably manage. (Your *intention* to treat a particular part of your back will activate the Reiki into that area.)

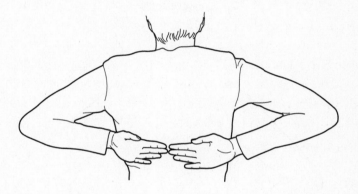

15b. As an alternative, you can place the back of each hand flat against your back, as high above your waist as you can comfortably manage.

16. THE WAIST

As well as covering the middle portion of the spine, and flowing into the solar plexus and sacral chakras, this hand position enables Reiki to flow again into some important organs such as the pancreas, digestive system, liver, kidneys, spleen and adrenal glands. The waist is also where our bodies bend physically, so metaphysically this area can show whether we are rigid and resentful, or flexible and accepting in our attitudes; whether we can adequately balance our own needs with others' demands. Whichever alternative hand position you adopt, hold it for between three and five minutes.

103

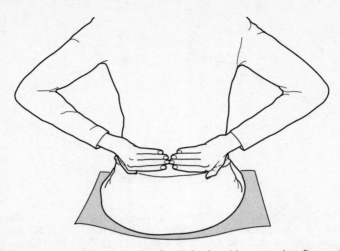

16a. Place one hand on each side of your body, with your palms flat against your back, fingers pointing toward each other, and thumbs tucked into your natural waistline.

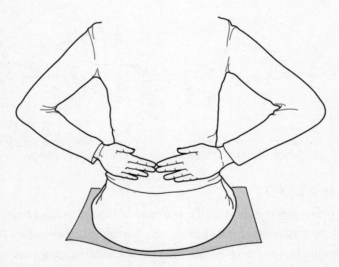

16b. Alternatively, place the back of each hand flat against your back, with the fingertips pointing toward each other, this time with your little finger tucked into your natural waistline.

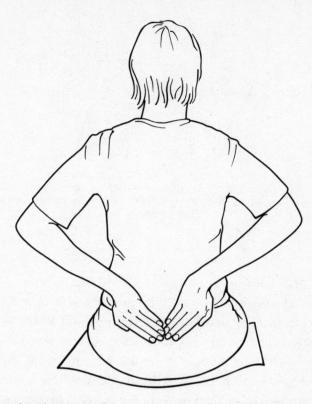

16c. As another alternative, you can place your hands with the heel of each hand at waist level and the fingertips pointing slightly downward in a V shape. (You can also do this as an extra hand position, if you have lower back pain.)

17. THE BUTTOCKS

This hand position covers the base chakra again, and the lower portion of the spine, including the coccyx, and therefore the skeleton, skin, blood and elimination system, as well as the genitals, testes, hips, legs and feet. However, the buttocks are also where we can "sit on" our feelings, especially fears of a lack of something, whether it be of a material or emotional nature; there are parental issues linked with this, as we tend to internalize our parents' expectations. Sometimes we can develop extra weight in this area as another way of smothering our real feelings or hiding our fears.

105

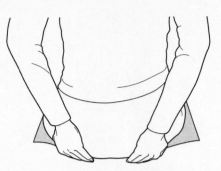

Place one hand on each buttock—it does not matter which way the hands are facing as long as it is comfortable, and hold your hands there for between three and five minutes.

The Legs and Feet

Our legs and feet connect us with the ground, carry us and move us forward in life, enabling us to walk, run, skip or climb, as well as to stand still, so problems here often relate to resistance or reluctance to move in a particular direction, or a fear of the future. We can live life "taking two steps forward and one step back," so that we delay getting what we want out of life, or we can be afraid of "running before we can walk"; or we can "get a move on" and live our lives to the full. Many of the "fun" things in life rely on our ability to use our legs and feet (dancing and most sports are examples), so problems here can relate to a lack of belief in our abilities, or even feeling that we don't deserve to enjoy life.

The illustrations below show each hand positioned on top of the thigh, knee, and so on, but you can place your hands underneath the thigh or knee, and on the calf instead of the shin, for a change sometimes. If any of the illustrated hand positions are difficult for you, it is OK to adjust the way you place your hands on your legs/feet, or adopt a different sitting position, or draw your legs up closer to your body so that you can comfortably hold the position for a few minutes.

Alternatively, if you are working on some specific issues relating to your direction in life, you can treat each leg separately, placing one hand above and one below each hand position, on the thigh, knee, lower leg, ankle and foot. (The following illustration shows an example of treating the knee in this way.)

106

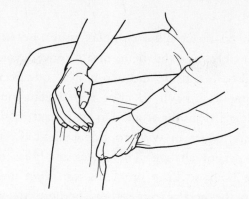

You can place one hand underneath and one hand on top of one knee at a time.

18. THE THIGHS

Deep issues from our past, particularly from our childhood, can be stored in our thighs. They include family matters and problems with our parents, questions of sex and sexuality, and old feelings of anger or resentment. These issues can be "locked up" in our thighs, and often reveal themselves in excess weight in this area.

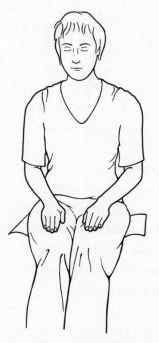

Place one hand on the top of each thigh for between one and two minutes.

107

19. THE KNEES

The knees can be about quite complex issues, because they allow us to move flexibly, to stand firm, or to concede or give way, so they are linked to our pride and ego and to our decision making. Are you finding it difficult to choose between your options, or afraid of making a decision at all? Do you react to situations with stubbornness and anger, or with confidence and assertiveness and a willingness to accept change? The knees also bear the load from the rest of the body, so knee problems can often indicate that we have "come to the end of our tether" because we simply cannot bear any more.

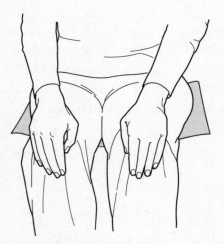

Place one hand on each knee for between one and two minutes.

20. THE SHINS AND CALVES

The lower part of the leg is about both our standing in life, and our resistance to or fear of moving forward in life, to a particular decision we have made or need to make, or to a specific life-path direction we have taken or need to take. Problems in this area often occur because we are trying to follow someone else's wishes (for example, those of a parent or partner), rather than our own.

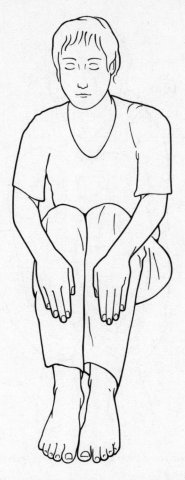

Place one hand on each shin for between one and two minutes.

21. THE ANKLES

The ankles are also about directions and willingness to move forward, and particularly about our ability to accept change and "go with the flow." If we are feeling nervous about changes in direction or lifestyle, then problems with our ankles can follow. In addition, the ankles support us when we stand or walk, so health problems here can be linked to whether we feel we get enough support from people around us, or whether we adequately support ourselves by our own actions.

109

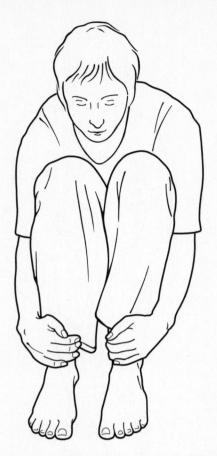

Place one hand on each ankle for one to two minutes.

22. THE FEET AND TOES

There are many phrases in our language that indicate how our feet are important to us, such as being able to "stand on your own two feet," meaning being independent and not having to rely on others, or "putting your best foot forward," meaning stepping confidently into our next task or direction. We use our feet to connect to the real world, and to journey through life, so problems with the feet can indicate distress about what is happening in the present, or fear of what might happen in the future. In a similar way, problems with the toes show worry about minor details. Whichever of the following hand positions you choose, hold it for one or two minutes.

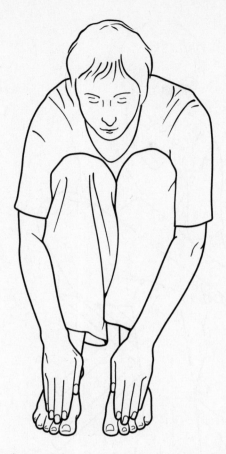

22a. Place one hand on each foot, so that your fingers also cover the toes.

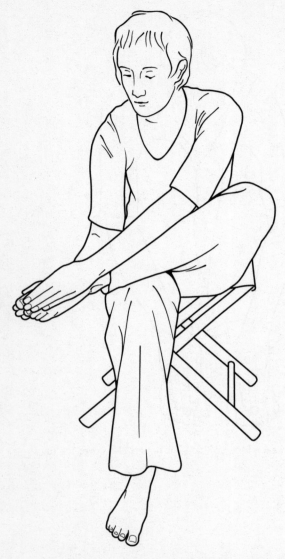

22b. Alternatively, place each hand underneath each foot, covering the sole.

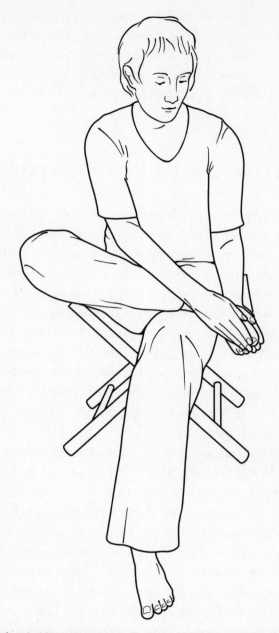

22c. The feet hold meridian points leading to all parts of the body, so to allow Reiki to flow once again around the whole body you can treat each foot separately, with one hand on top and one underneath the foot. It doesn't matter which foot you treat first. Hold each foot for between one and two minutes.

At the end of your self-treatment, place your hands again in position 1 on the crown of your head (*see diagram on page 87*) and *intend* that Reiki now closes your energy field. Afterward I usually place my hands in the *Gassho* position and breathe deeply, allowing myself to become centered again and giving thanks to Reiki.

PERSONALIZING YOUR SELF-TREATMENT

The above hand positions and timings are given as a framework, but as you get more practice with Reiki you will find yourself drawn to change things sometimes, and that's fine. Reiki will work with you to enhance your intuition and self-awareness, and you need to develop trust in your own responses, to how you feel during the treatment, rather than just slavishly following a set of instructions every time. For example, the amount of time you spend in each hand position doesn't have to be exactly as I have suggested. Three to five minutes on a head or body hand position is a good average to aim for, but if you feel you need ten or fifteen minutes, then take that time. Similarly, if you sense that part of you has received enough Reiki in less than three minutes, simply move on.

It makes sense to treat any part of you that is sore or injured for longer, but you might also feel that it is a good idea to keep your hands longer on parts of you that relate to any issues you are working with at the time. For each of the above hand positions, I have put forward some ideas about what they are treating not only on a physical level, but also on causative levels. For instance, if you feel you would like to develop greater self-esteem and belief in yourself, or if you are finding it hard to "stomach" what is going on around you, then treating the solar plexus for longer would be a good idea. Similarly, if you find it difficult to speak openly, especially in public, or cannot express your emotions effectively even to your partner, you could find treating your neck and throat chakra for longer very beneficial.

The point is that self-healing is a very personal thing, and therefore a self-treatment is also very personal and you can tailor it to your specific needs. You can treat yourself for many hours at a time if you are really ill, or fit in a quick treatment in your lunch break in order to de-stress yourself at work. You can create a program of treatments to work on specific physical problems or personal issues, spending longer on one or two hand positions and shortening the others, and so on. Self-treatments are a part of treating yourself well in your everyday life, so sometimes you will want to pamper yourself while at other times you'll just need a quick "touch-up." Just use your common sense and enjoy the fact that you have at your fingertips—literally—a tool for helping yourself to better health and greater well-being.

THE EFFECTS OF SELF-TREATMENT

So what can you expect of self-treatment with Reiki? Unfortunately, the answer to that is the same as the answer to "how long is a piece of string?" because it all depends! It depends upon what physical, emotional, mental or spiritual issues you are dealing with on both a conscious and a subconscious level, because Reiki will be working on all levels whenever you use it for self-treatment.

Because Reiki is actually your own Soul energy, working in harmony with your whole body and whole self, it will always work for your highest and greatest good, but that doesn't mean that the effects will always be pleasant, at least in the short term. For example, when I began experimenting with the "Whole Body, Whole Self" treatment, at first it just felt very pleasant and even more relaxing than usual. After about a week I noticed a great increase in the heat I felt in my hands when I was treating my arms and legs, and soon I went through a "healing crisis," meaning that distressing symptoms began to arise as the Reiki dislodged some of the layers of blockage that I had been holding on to for a long time.

With me, those symptoms were stiff and painful knees, and even stiffer and more painful hands and fingers. Not pleasant, and very inconvenient, since I was actually writing this book at the time and needed to sit at a computer and operate a keyboard every day! But

115

I persevered with the self-treatments, and gradually insights began to occur to me into the reasons for the exaggerated symptoms, although at first I found them quite difficult to accept. I will share them with you, because I think they will show you just how valuable this type of "body language" can be. Basically they revealed that, at a deep level, I was actually afraid of writing this book, and very fearful of the responsibility I was taking on and the direction it was taking me in. Does that surprise you? Well, it surprised me! I love teaching Reiki, and I love writing and putting the two together has until now been a very joyful experience. But writing this book was taking me to a different level both personally and professionally.

Firstly, there was the perhaps natural hesitation I felt about writing about self-healing when I hadn't personally achieved it—or rather, when I hadn't personally achieved supreme good health and a totally "sorted" life. But then I'm human, not superhuman; and as I've said earlier in this book, I am on my own personal healing journey, just like everyone else. The fact that I've been self-treating with Reiki for more than twenty years means that Reiki is now able to reach ever-deeper levels of blockage and resistance. The result of this is that sometimes for short periods my health is actually worse than it was a few years ago—but that only means it is going through stages of getting a bit worse before it gets better, as I let go of old blocked emotions and old thought patterns that are holding me back.

Once I recognize what is going on, I actively go through the self-healing process of acknowledgment, acceptance, awareness and action (*see page 29*), working on whatever issue the healing has brought up for me to look at, and then the symptoms subside again, sometimes slowly, sometimes quickly. Or sometimes they don't disappear, and I realize there is more work to do, so I continue with my daily self-treatments, knowing that eventually I will intuitively reach an understanding. And then I let go of it. I don't worry about how long it will take before I'm "better." It will take as long as it needs.

Let me remind you again—I am human, so sometimes I do find it frustrating, and of course I want to be physically fit, healthy and vibrantly well all the time. Everyone wants that. As a Reiki Master, however, I realize that I have chosen to be on a very conscious journey of self-realization and self-mastery, so sometimes I have to recognize that an illness is a lesson in itself—that it is not about getting rid of it, but about learning to live with it and, even harder, learning to love it.

Hmmm. OK, that's a tough one—and if you're going through health problems that are difficult to live with I know you'll understand, and I empathize with your problems, too. But at least my belief system—that everything has a purpose—allows me to be more accepting and more positive about ill health. I don't feel a "victim" of it. I feel potentially empowered by it, because I recognize that it is another learning opportunity—and if that makes me sound a bit pious, I apologize! I'm no saint, I assure you, and I'm as ready as anyone else to rant about the unfairness of it all sometimes, but the point is that I know that eventually I will realize the gift the illness has given me.

That gift may be a greater understanding of a particular issue I'm working through, or the realization that I need to treat my body better by changing my diet, or the motivation to change direction or do something different to bring more joy into my life. There are always benefits, but I will admit that they are usually only seen with hindsight, and hindsight, as we all know, is 20/20 vision!

As I finish this chapter, I'm pleased to report that, having faced up to my fears and having asked my Higher Self for guidance, I have decided to rewrite certain sections of the book that I wasn't really happy with, and my hands and knees are beginning to feel more flexible again, so I guess I have uncovered what I needed to uncover for the moment—until the next time!

As you can see, the answer to the question I posed at the beginning of this section, "What can you expect of a Reiki self-treatment?" can be multidimensional, but it is always, always, beneficial and for your highest and greatest good. And of course there are some immediate benefits from a self-treatment, such as a sense of deep relaxation, being able to sleep better, feeling calm and better able to cope with life's ups and downs and so on.

SELF-TREATMENT AS A MEDITATION

To enhance your self-treatment still further, you might like to try this exercise. As you place your hands in the first position, begin to breathe deeply and evenly, *intending* that with each in-breath you are breathing in Reiki, and with each out-breath you are letting go of any energetic impurities from your energy body. This takes some concentration, and turns the self-treatment into a form of meditation. As soon as you can, let each in-breath take about three seconds, and each out-breath also take about three seconds. This will gradually slow your heart rate, and as you become more and more relaxed and take in more and more Reiki with each breath, you will probably find that your inhalations and exhalations become stronger and slower, taking five seconds each or even longer. However, unless you are very practiced at deep meditation, nine seconds is probably the maximum you should aim for—any longer and you can become light-headed instead of light-filled, due to lack of oxygen!

USING THE SYMBOLS FOR SELF-TREATMENT

A traditional self-treatment, or the "Whole Body, Whole Self" treatment described above, can be made even more effective by using the Power Symbol if you have done Second Degree. Before you start, empower your whole energy field by drawing a Power Symbol on each palm, and a large Power Symbol in front of your whole body, silently saying its mantra three times each time you use it. Then, before placing your hands in each of the hand positions, visualize a Power Symbol either in the air above, or directly on the body in the area that is being treated, each time silently saying its mantra three times.

A MENTAL AND EMOTIONAL SELF-TREATMENT

A particularly effective way of carrying out a self-treatment is to include the special "mental and emotional" treatment taught at Second Degree. You can begin either the traditional twelve-hand-position self-treatment or the "Whole Body, Whole Self" treatment in this way, and it doesn't take very long once you have practiced it a few times. You do need to maintain concentration for about five minutes while you carry out the visualization, but afterward you can shorten the length of time you spend on the other hand positions, if you wish. It begins with a different hand position, where your nondominant hand (usually your left) is placed at the back of your head, and your dominant hand is then free to draw the symbols over your crown, after which it is placed on the top of your head (*see illustration below*). It is probably easiest to do this treatment while lying down, so that your hands and arms are well supported, but it can be done in a sitting position.

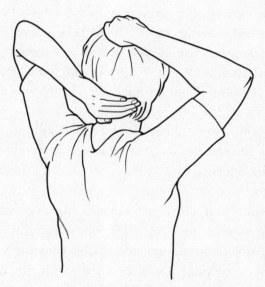

Mental and emotional self-treatment hand position.

1. Start by sitting or lying quietly with your hands on your heart chakra, doing Reiki on yourself for a few moments.

2. Draw a large Power Symbol from the top of your head down to your base chakra so as to clear, protect and empower you, silently saying its sacred mantra three times. (Remember at all times that the Reiki symbols are sacred, and you should ensure that no one else can see the symbols being drawn or hear their mantras.)

3. Next, draw the Power Symbol on each of your palms; say its mantra three times, then place one hand under the back of your head so that it covers the occipital bone.

4. With the other hand draw all three symbols over your crown chakra, starting with the Distant Symbol, saying its sacred mantra three times, and then saying your own name three times.

5. Draw the Harmony Symbol, say the mantra three times and your name three times.

6. Finally, draw the Power Symbol, say the mantra three times, and imagine each symbol going through the crown, brow and throat chakras and into the heart. Think, believe and *intend* that this Reiki energy is channeled with love and light for your highest and greatest good to create deep healing on all levels—physical, mental, emotional and spiritual.

7. When you have finished this, place the hand that you have used to draw the symbols on your crown chakra, and begin the visualization sequence.

8. Now with your inner eye, visualize Reiki as soft white light flowing out of the palm of your dominant hand on the crown of your head, until it is filling your head, and then see or sense it swirling slowly down through the whole of your body—into the neck and shoulders, down each arm, into the chest, waist and abdomen, into the hips and legs, right down to the toes. When you can visualize your whole body completely filled with soft white light, leaving the white light filling your whole body, slowly turn your attention back to the palm of your hand, which is resting on your crown chakra.

9. Imagine that Reiki, as a rainbow of colored light (which may be composed of all seven colors, or just a few—whatever you see is right for you at this moment) is flowing out of the palm of

your hand until it fills your head. Slowly take this rainbow of colored light through your whole body right down to your fingers and toes, then, leaving the rainbow light filling your whole body, allow your visioning to come back once more to the hand covering your crown chakra.

10. Visualize Reiki as brilliant, sparkling white light flowing out of your palm, becoming brighter and brighter, and imagine this brilliant white light once more flowing through the whole of your head and body, until every part of you is completely filled with brilliant, sparkling white light.

11. As soon as your body is filled with this brilliant white light, imagine the light spreading out of your physical body to fill the whole of your aura. Imagine it flowing into the first layer, and when that is full, see it spilling over into the second layer, and then on into the third layer, and then the fourth layer and the fifth layer. Sense it spilling over into the sixth layer and then on into the seventh layer, so that the whole of your aura is filled with shimmering, sparkling white light.

12. Next, imagine the brilliant white light expanding still further, until it flows out beyond your aura, swirling upward and outward until it fills the whole room with Reiki as sparkling white light.

13. Now visualize a strand of that Reiki, as brilliant white light, coming up out of your solar plexus chakra or heart chakra (or both). In your imagination take the strand of brilliant white light, still connected to your body, and let it lengthen until it goes through the ceiling, and then stretches up above the building, right up into the sky, and then higher and higher, through the clouds and up into the blue sky beyond, until it reaches the very edge of the Earth's atmosphere.

14. Pause for a moment, and let the strand of Reiki white light gradually expand outward. See it growing and spreading out across

and around the whole world, sense it meeting up with other strands of Reiki light until the whole world is covered in a fine mesh of Reiki, holding the Earth in a web of healing.

15. Take your attention back to that narrow beam of Reiki light, and let it flow up beyond the Earth's atmosphere, further and further through space, past the stars, heading toward the center of the Universe, toward the Light, the Source, the All-That-Is. Feel it connect with the ultimate Source of all love, and all light, and all healing, and sense some of that love and light and healing flowing back down that strand of Reiki light. This ultimate unconditional love and deep healing may appear like liquid golden light, or like a soft blue smoke, or it may be of any other color. Gradually it will flow down the strand of Reiki light, back through space, back through the Earth's atmosphere, back down through the sky, through the roof and the ceiling and into your body. Visualize and sense that love, light and deep healing flooding throughout your body, until every part is completely filled with this beautiful, peaceful, loving energy.

16. When you intuitively sense that this process is complete, slowly take your attention back up to where the strand of Reiki light is connected to the Source, and with a sense of gratitude and respect gently detach the strand and begin to bring that narrow beam of Reiki back down through space, through the Earth's atmosphere, through the ceiling, until it is once more inside your body.

17. When you have completed the visualization, seal in this special healing by drawing a Power Symbol over your solar plexus chakra and/or heart chakra, saying the mantra three times, and *intending* that this unconditional love and deep healing be sealed into your body.

18. Finally, take your dominant hand off your head and draw the Power Symbol once more in the air over your crown chakra. Say the mantra three times, with the *intention* of closing your chakras and ending the Mental and Emotional part of the treatment.

Closing this part of the treatment properly is as important for you in a self-treatment as it is when using this type of treatment on another person. It seals in the Reiki and closes the crown chakra, which means that you can then reduce your level of concentration. You can, of course, end with a statement of gratitude to Reiki for its many blessings and healing.

You can now continue your self-treatment in the normal way, placing your hands in each of the twenty-two hand positions in the "Whole Body, Whole Self" treatment above, or the twelve hand positions of a traditional self-treatment, but you can reduce the time for each position to about half if you wish, as your whole being has already been permeated with Reiki.

SENDING A DISTANT TREATMENT TO YOURSELF

The techniques taught at Second Degree level enable you to send very powerful healing to anyone, anywhere, at any time, including in the past and in the future—and that includes being able to send a Reiki treatment to yourself! Using the Distant (Connection) Symbol allows you to connect to any person (or animal) to whom you wish to send healing, forming a "bridge" that cuts through time and space, and along which the Reiki can flow. This means that you can carry out a distant treatment on yourself and "program" it for some later time, when you know you will be able to lie down and receive it, rather like setting a video recorder to record a favorite program, and then sitting down at a convenient time to watch it. You can even "program" a number of Reiki treatments to go to you, for example each night while you are asleep for the next seven nights. (After seven treatments it is best to redo the distant treatment as it seems to lose some strength over time, but you can then reprogram it for another seven nights, if you wish.)

You can place your hands directly on your own body, or use a photograph of yourself, or write your name (and address) on a piece of paper and hold that between your hands, or just visualize yourself.

You can also use a "correspondence"—something that you can use to represent yourself, such as a teddy bear or even a pillow, so you have something to place your hands on. The process is quite simple, and you can either do a standard distant treatment, where you use the Distant Symbol and the Power Symbol, or a Mental and Emotional distant treatment, where you use the Harmony Symbol as well.

1. Draw the Distant Symbol over your crown chakra, or over the photo, paper or body of the correspondence. Say its mantra three times, your name three times and your location once (for example "my bedroom at 17 Acacia Avenue, Anytown").

2. If you intend to carry out a Mental and Emotional treatment, draw the Harmony Symbol next over your crown chakra or over the photo, paper or body of the correspondence. Say its mantra three times and your name once. (If you are intending to do a standard distant treatment, leave out this step.)

3. Next, draw a Power Symbol over your crown chakra, or over the photo, paper or body of the correspondence, and say its mantra three times. Then say, "This Reiki treatment (or this Reiki Mental and Emotional treatment) is to be received by me at (time and date you have decided) or (when I am asleep tonight) or even (when it will be most beneficial)."

4. If you are carrying out a distant Mental and Emotional self-treatment, you then start the visualization, imagining the soft white light of Reiki flowing through you, and so on (*see pages 118–23 for the whole sequence*). Remember to end by drawing another Power Symbol over your crown chakra, *intending* to seal in the healing and end the Mental and Emotional part of the treatment.

5. You can then carry out a standard treatment by placing your hands as if they were in each of the twelve (or twenty-two) hand positions, for one or two minutes each, either actually on your own body, or on the correspondence or in the air above a photo, and so on.

If you are intending to program a number of treatments, when you reach step three above replace the instruction with the following: "This Reiki is to be received by me at (time decided upon) or (when I am asleep) today (or tonight) and for the following six days (or nights)." Then, after one week, you can either get back to doing the Distant Treatment on a daily basis, or if the same conditions still exist for you, you can reprogram the treatment for another seven days.

In the next chapter there are some ideas for other ways of treating yourself with Reiki, including alternatives to holding your hands still in the same place.

chapter 6

OTHER METHODS OF SELF-TREATMENT

Although doing a self-treatment every day is an excellent practice to promote self-healing, it isn't the only way to give yourself Reiki. Reiki can be as flexible as you are, so you can place your hands anywhere on your body and allow the energy to flow through you almost anywhere, at any time, throughout the day. You can add to your daily self-treatment as often as you like, giving yourself five or ten minutes of Reiki, or longer if you want, by just placing your hands on an appropriately convenient place—your chest, solar plexus, stomach or thighs are usually the easiest—and intending that Reiki should flow for your highest and greatest good.

The point is that if you have some time to spare, use it to give yourself Reiki. It doesn't require any conscious effort on your part. You don't even *have* to be sitting or lying down. Simply put your hands on any part of your body that you can comfortably reach and allow the Reiki to flow. You can do this while you are watching television, sitting at the movies, waiting at a bus stop or relaxing in the staff lounge after lunch. Because your hands will simply be lying still somewhere on your body, no one will be any the wiser if you don't want to reveal what you are doing.

GIVING YOURSELF "FIRST AID" TREATMENT

There is no need to give yourself a full self-treatment every time you have a headache, bang your elbow or cut your finger. Although a full self-treatment is always beneficial it isn't always essential, so if you have a stiff neck or aching shoulders, a headache or sore eyes, treat them individually. All you need to do is *intend* that the Reiki should flow, and it will. If your injury is more serious, it makes sense to seek medical help or advice—although you can give yourself Reiki while you wait for professional attention (but note the cautions below).

As well as giving yourself Reiki for first aid, remember to give yourself lots of Reiki if you are ill. You cannot "overdose" on Reiki, so if you are feeling ill just place your hands on yourself anywhere that is comfortable, and let the Reiki flow for as many hours as you like. It will accelerate your body's own healing processes, mobilizing your immune system to heal wounds faster, or fight off whatever "bug" you have caught. Initially it may be a little uncomfortable, and it may even exacerbate your symptoms, because many of the distressing symptoms we experience when we are ill or injured are actually the effects of the body's activities to fight off infection, release toxins or accelerate cell growth to close wounds, but it will shorten the length of time you feel ill, which has to be a good thing.

TIMES FOR CAUTION

You rarely need to exercise caution when giving Reiki, but there are a couple of issues to look out for. If you are unlucky enough to accidentally chop off a toe or finger, for example, the obvious thing to do is to pack the missing part carefully and get to a hospital as quickly as possible so that it can be reattached surgically.

The caution here relates to the fact that Reiki accelerates your body's own healing ability—if you applied Reiki directly to the hand or foot in this case, the natural healing process would quickly begin to take place and the wound could heal too rapidly to allow the missing digit to be reattached. I know of at least one case where a severed finger could not be reattached even though the man in question went straight to hospital after the accident. The medical staff could not understand why he had not come to the hospital sooner, as the wound had healed so much that it looked as though the accident had happened several days before. (Because Reiki always works for your highest and greatest good, you may be questioning why this happened, but we cannot know how that man's highest good was served. Maybe it was a form of "wake-up call" to get him to change career, for instance.)

By all means give yourself Reiki in cases such as this—just don't apply it directly on the injured part. Instead, place a hand on your heart chakra or over your kidneys to help with the pain and shock. Although the Reiki will flow throughout the body, including to the injury, it will do so in a much gentler way, so the healing effect will not be so dramatic.

The same caution applies in the case of a bad break of an arm, leg, wrist or ankle. This will probably need professional setting, and again, if the healing process has already begun this could cause problems, because the bone(s) might not be aligned properly. Apply Reiki to your heart chakra or adrenal glands to deal with the pain and shock rather than placing your hand directly on the break. After the bone has been set and plastered, give it as much Reiki as possible—it will mend more quickly.

Potentially, Reiki can heal broken bones within hours. A friend of mine, also a Reiki Master, broke several bones in her hand and worked on it with another Reiki Master. Within hours all the bruising and swelling had gone, and by the next day her hand was so well healed that she was able to carry out several aromatherapy massages. However, working in this way does take a great deal of belief in Reiki and trust in its process, and the instance I have quoted may have happened in the way it did just to prove that it was possible. Under normal circumstances, I would always advise people to get a broken bone properly set.

SOME QUICK AND EASY TREATMENTS

Quick Energy Boosts

Sometimes when your energy is running low because you have been busy or had a stressful day, you could do with a bit of a boost. I have come up with this technique, which seems to work well.

The Ten-minute Touch-up

1. First, *intend* that the Reiki should flow for your highest and greatest good (just thinking that you want to use Reiki will activate it). Place one hand over your eyes, with the palm facing and touching your face, and the other hand at the back of your head, palm against the head. (It doesn't matter which hand is where: for instance the left hand can be at the front or back.) Hold your hands in this position for two and a half minutes—counting to 150 is the way I keep a check on the time, but of course you can look at a clock, or even carry on for longer if you want to.

2. Next, place one hand on your throat and the other on the center of your chest, again for about two and a half minutes.

3. Then place one hand on your solar plexus and the other on your navel for another two and a half minutes.

4. Finally, place one hand on the top of your head, over your crown chakra, and the other on your root chakra, either on your bottom (or underneath it if you are sitting down), or with your hand between your legs for two and a half minutes.

The "Wake-up"

This hand position works well as a quick "wake-up," when you are feeling tired but need to carry on with some tasks, and it is also good for hangovers (although rehydrating your body by drinking plenty of water would probably be even better!). Place both hands, one hand crossed over the other, on the crown of your head as you would in the self-treatment hand position shown on page 87. *Intend* that the Reiki should flow, and keep your hands in that position for at least five minutes, or until you are feeling better.

The Back Treatment

If you have a bad back there is a particular hand position that you might find helpful, although it does mean you have to be flexible enough to place your hands behind you. Put one hand (it doesn't matter which) at the top of your neck, just below the base of your skull, and place the other on your coccyx (roughly where you sit down). Let the Reiki flow for at least five minutes. If holding the position for long is painful, feel free to change hands around whenever you need to.

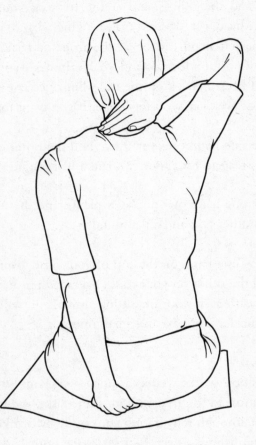

Treatment for a bad back.

A Quick Self-treatment Using Symbols

I'm not suggesting that this method should be used frequently in place of a full self-treatment, but it is excellent when you are short of time, or just wish to give yourself a "renewal" of energy. Using the symbols enhances the amount of Reiki you can receive in a short time, so if you have Second Degree doing this for about five minutes is probably equivalent to at least ten minutes of a traditional self-treatment.

1. Hold out your hands in front of you and envision yourself between them. (You can use a piece of paper with your name on it, or a photograph of yourself.) With your dominant hand, draw the Distant Symbol over your other hand, silently saying its mantra three times and your own name three times.

2. Draw the Harmony Symbol over your hand/name/photo, silently saying its mantra three times and your own name three times.

3. Draw the Power Symbol over your hand/name/photo, silently saying its mantra three times.

4. Hold your dominant hand over your other hand/name/photo, and intend that Reiki should flow to you for your greatest and highest good. Maintain this position for five to ten minutes, or for as long as you wish.

5. Draw the Power Symbol over your hand/name/photo again, saying its mantra three times and *intending* that this wonderful healing energy be sealed in; *intend* that the treatment is over.

OTHER WAYS OF USING THE HANDS WITH REIKI

Most people who do Reiki are only used to holding their hands flat and still when treating themselves or others. In the Japanese tradition there were other methods of using the hands to provide additional stimulation with Reiki on the physical body. These methods are particularly useful for areas where you have found energetic disturbances when you have scanned your body before treatment (*see page 79*). Obviously, you would not use these techniques on any sore or sensitive parts of your body. As always, while carrying out these techniques you should *intend* that the Reiki will flow through your hands (palms and fingertips) for your highest and greatest good.

The Japanese names of these techniques all use the word *Te*, meaning "hand," and end in *Chiryo-ho*, which means "medical treatment or method."

Uchi-te Chiryo-ho

Uchi means "to strike, hit, knock or pound," and this is therefore a technique for patting with the hands (gently, although the translation of *uchi* makes it sound like battering!). It is ideal for use on areas of numbness, or where energy feels stagnant and blocked, as it encourages greater energy flow and movement.

Using a firm but gentle motion (not hard enough to hurt), use the flat of your hand (palm and fingers flat) to pat and stimulate the area, starting with very soft patting and gradually making it a bit stronger, so that the motion becomes a soft slapping. Continue until you sense that it is time to move to another position (probably after between thirty seconds and a minute). This treatment will stimulate the surface of the physical body and enable Reiki to penetrate into your body quickly, waking up the cells and breaking up any energy blockages.

Nade-te Chiryo-ho

Nade means "to stroke, pat or smooth down," and stroking with the hands while using Reiki encourages your body's own energies to flow smoothly, as well as promoting a greater flow of Reiki so that it can penetrate your body easily and quickly. It feels very comforting and soothing, and of course when you're treating yourself you can use this method while dressed or undressed. The action is gentle surface stroking, not massage.

Place your hands flat on your body, starting on any part you choose. Gently, but with an acceptably firm pressure to avoid tickling yourself, stroke your hands in a downward direction (for example from the shoulder down the arm to the hand) in short movements of about five to ten centimeters (two to four inches), or in small circles, encouraging the energy flow with Reiki and giving gentle stimulation with the friction of your hands.

Oshi-te Chiryo-ho

Oshi means "push or pressure," so this is a method of using slight pressure with your fingertips, pushing them gently but firmly into areas such as stiff or aching muscles, or places where there is some numbness or a feeling of energy blockage or stagnation, and allowing the Reiki to flow and gently stimulate the area to activate healing. Don't press too hard, and you will obviously find this technique more pleasant if you have reasonably short nails rather than long ones.

You don't have to use all your fingers for this technique. You generally use only two fingers on each hand, or on one hand only. It is probably easiest to use either the index and middle fingers, or the middle and ring fingers, or even the tips of your thumbs on the area which is stiff or where you detect a blockage. Gently apply a little pressure, intending that Reiki will flow through the fingers to treat that area and/or break up energy blockages. To loosen particularly stubborn stiff shoulders or aching muscles, gently vibrate or rotate your fingers/thumbs backward and forward slightly, sending Reiki through the fingertips.

THE JAPANESE NAVEL TREATMENT

In Eastern medicine the navel is regarded as a very important point in the body, both energetically and physically. Just below the navel is the site of the sacral chakra, which is sometimes called the Tan-dien point, or the Hara, and this is regarded as the energy center of the body and therefore the most important point for healing any illness or disease. This technique from the Japanese tradition is called *Heso Chiryo-ho*—*Heso* means navel, *Chiryo* means medical treatment, and *Ho* is treatment, method or way—and it is a method for balancing the flow of Ki in the body to promote healing.

Start by sitting or standing in a comfortable position, and spend a few moments breathing deeply and evenly to center yourself, with your hands in the *Gassho* position. When you feel calm, *intend* that the Reiki should flow into you to promote deep healing for your greatest and highest good. Then place one hand (usually your dominant hand) against your body, with your middle finger inserted into your navel, ensuring that you can feel your own pulse—and by that I mean your energetic pulse, not the pulse from the aorta, which can also be detected at a deeper level at this point. (If you can feel that pulse, you're pushing your finger in too hard.) You can place your other hand elsewhere on the body, for instance over your heart chakra, if you wish. Sense and *intend* that your energetic pulse is resonating in harmony with Reiki, and hold this position until you feel relaxed and balanced, which will probably take about five to ten minutes. Then remove your finger from your navel and spend another few minutes quietly resting before resuming other activities.

Hopefully, chapters 5 and 6 have given you lots of ideas on how to use Reiki for self-treatment. In Part III you will find a wide range of other suggestions for using Reiki to heal your whole self, from your energy body and physical body to your emotional, mental and spiritual self.

part three

HEALING YOUR WHOLE
SELF

chapter 7

HEALING YOUR ENERGY BODY

The aura, chakras and meridians that carry life-force energy (Ki) and make up the human energy body are very important elements in the health of any individual, because it is the blockages and damage that occur in the energy body which can manifest eventually as physical illness or disease if they are not cleared and healed. As I mentioned in Chapter 3, the human energy field is energy vibrating at a high rate, so it is lighter and finer than the physical body, which is why other high-energy vibrations affect it, such as mental or thought energy, emotional energy, and electromagnetic energy like radio waves and cell phone signals. Basically, everything that happens to you—both negative and positive experiences—affects your energy body, although of course it is the negative experiences that create the blockages and eventual damage. In this chapter I discuss how we can heal the whole energy body, but I would like to begin with an examination of the aura.

WHAT AFFECTS THE AURA?

The aura, a field of light around your physical body, reflects your overall health and well-being, and some very psychic people, who are often called "medical intuitives," are able to detect many different kinds of imbalance within the aura. Illness and disease appear there first, usually as dark, "sticky" or "muddy" patches of denser energy. These can collect in any of the seven layers of the aura, but the closer they get to the physical body the more likely it is that the energy will become dense enough to transform into physical matter or into elements that can affect physical matter. When these blockages appear very close to any of the major chakras, it usually means that they are about to make the transformation into the physical, so in a later section we will be looking at ways of dispersing energy at that level.

What actually affects the aura? Mental energy, or thought energy, including the spoken word, is one potential hazard. Every negative thought you have ever had, every negative word you have spoken, will have had an effect on the aura, although sometimes the effect will be quite transient. Generally any negative effects would normally only be lasting if the negative thoughts and words were consistently repeated. Similarly, any negative words spoken to you or negative actions performed toward you can potentially form damaging energy patterns in your aura, as can reading the newspapers, which are usually filled with negative news, or watching violent or horror films or television programs. These all have a dampening effect on your energy field, lowering your energy body's vibrations, or life force. To balance things out your energies are also affected by positive mental energy, so when you are praised, succeed with a creative project, have some success at work, read positive news or watch a comedy that makes you laugh out loud, your energies are raised and you feel good.

Emotional energy also affects the aura: when you experience negative emotions such as anger, resentment, jealousy, hatred or fear, or have these emotions directed toward you by other people, they will have a bad effect on your energies. Fortunately, our lives are not constantly filled only with negative emotions, so the love and affection we gain from our family and friends, from watching children at play or from viewing a magnificent sunset, or the emotions raised by reading beautiful poetry or listening to wonderfully uplifting music, all have beneficial effects on the body's energy field. It is therefore usually only major traumas and significant or constantly repeated negative experiences that have the opportunity to damage our energy field beyond our normal ability to replenish and repair it.

Your energy field can additionally be affected negatively by other energies that are vibrating at a faster rate than your physical body, such as television and radio waves, cell phone signals, overhead electricity cables or substations, and so on, but I will be dealing with these in a later chapter.

YOUR LIFE-FORCE ENERGY—KI

Your aura and the rest of your energy body constitute your life-force energy, or Ki, and the idea that this energy exists has been part of the wisdom of most cultures around the world for many thousands of years. Taoist Master Ni Hua Ching describes Chi or Ki in this way:

> Chi (Ki) is the vital universal energy which composes,
> permeates and moves through everything that exists.
> Ki may be defined as the ultimate cause, and, at the
> same time, the ultimate effect.
> When Ki conglomerates, it is called matter.
> When Ki is diffuse, it is called space.
> When Ki animates form, it is called life.
> When Ki separates and withdraws from form, it is called death.
> When Ki flows, there is health.
> When Ki is blocked, there is sickness and disease.
> Ki embraces all things, circulates through and
> sustains them.

The amount of Ki within us does vary from day to day—there is a natural rhythmic ebb and flow in the energies within our bodies—but we absorb Ki in a variety of ways in order to "touch up" our supply of life force, because clearly we use some of it every day. The most obvious form in which we take in Ki is through food and drink, because all animal and plant life, and even water, is filled with this life-force energy too. We also breathe it in, and absorb it through our aura, as Ki energy is everywhere—it is the connective force of the Universe, so there is a limitless supply.

The amount of Ki we absorb is not constant, however, and can depend on many factors. We therefore don't always replenish our supply sufficiently, and if this happens over a long period of time our energy body can become too depleted. We then become weaker and more susceptible to illness and the aging process, and even to physical death—because your Ki, or life force, is what defines you as a living being, and without it you would not be alive. This means that when your Ki is high and flowing freely around your whole energy body, you feel healthy, strong, fit and full of energy, and also confident, ready to enjoy life and take on its challenges. When you feel like this, you are much less likely to become ill than if your Ki is low, or if there is a restriction or blockage in its flow; in the latter case you may feel weak, tired, listless and lethargic, and will therefore be much more vulnerable to illness, or "dis-ease."

The levels of life force in our bodies have an impact on our inherent healing ability, as Ki helps to nourish the structure, organs and systems of the body, supporting them in their vital functions and contributing to the healthy growth and renewal of cells. Since your aura is the outward expression of your life force, it makes sense to start your self-healing at this level.

CLEANSING YOUR AURA WITH REIKI

The most sensible place to start is with cleansing your aura, so refer to the various energy-cleansing techniques in Chapter 4. I would suggest using the Reiki shower and/or the *Kenyoku-ho* (*see pages 56–58 and 59–61*), or the whole of *Hatsurei-ho* (*see pages 58–64*) on a regular basis. You can then balance your aura with Reiki light, as follows.

1. Sit or stand comfortably, and place your hands in the *Gassho* position; spend a few moments breathing deeply and evenly, until you feel calm and centered.

2. Raise your hands above your head, palms facing each other, and *intend* that Reiki should begin flowing into your crown chakra. When you feel your palms or fingers begin to tingle with Reiki,

bring your arms down in an arc so that each palm is facing the sides
of your body, about sixty centimeters (two feet) away from you.

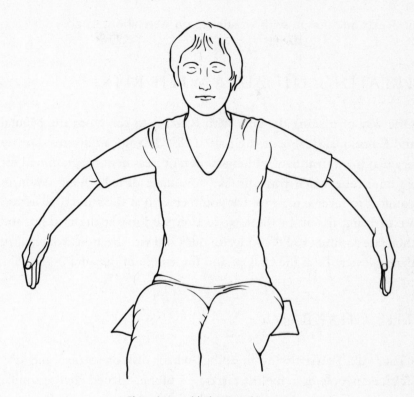

Cleansing and balancing the aura.

3. *Intend* that Reiki flows out of each palm to clear, balance and harmonize all the layers of your aura; you may like to visualize the
   Reiki as shimmering light, flowing out of each hand and swirling
   into and around your aura. You may intuitively sense areas of
   blockage in your aura, represented by darker patches that can be
   light or dark gray, brown or muddy yellow, and you may be able to
   "watch" as these begin to disperse as the Reiki works on them.

4. Remain in this position, showering Reiki into your aura, for
   between three and five minutes, or until you sense that your aura
   is filled with the vibrating, healing light of Reiki and any blockages have disappeared.

5. Place your hands once more in the *Gassho* position, and give thanks for the Reiki.

6. Relax and get on with whatever you were about to do.

TREATING THE AURA WITH REIKI

One way of treating the aura with Reiki is to carry out the Mental and Emotional treatment (*see pages 118–23*). You can do this directly as a hands-on treatment, either as a distant treatment programmed for a future time when you can take advantage of it by lying down in comfort to receive it, or so that you receive it at the same time as you are carrying it out. In the next section we look at the chakras, and there are a number of Reiki techniques and visualizations you can try that will treat both the chakras and the whole of the aura.

THE CHAKRAS

Chakra is a Sanskrit word meaning "wheel, disk or vortex," and very intuitive people describe the chakras as funnel-shaped energy, similar to a tornado or a whirlpool, with the narrowest point near the body and the widest visible point between thirty and sixty centimeters (one to two feet) away from the body. The chakras are points of intersection between the physical and the metaphysical planes, so they are effectively where mind and body meet. Whatever a chakra encounters on its particular vibrational level gets drawn into it, processed and passed out again, so this is where negative, dense energy can be drawn into the physical body to manifest on the physical plane as illness or disease.

The seven major chakras, in particular, are affected and shaped by our thoughts, emotions, experiences and the repeated patterns and actions in our daily lives, as well as by programming or patterning from our parents and other significant people, the culture and situations we are born into, our physical body shape, and even (if you are prepared to believe in reincarnation) unresolved patterns from previous lives. In some Hindu myths, chakras are seen as a kind of discus, thrown out only to come back to us, like a boomerang, hence the idea of karma, which postulates that the sum of a person's actions in previous lives decides their fate in future lives.

This is one explanation for becoming trapped in self-perpetuating action, which keeps us "stuck" in a chakra—we are caught in a pattern or archetype that keeps us at a particular level. If the patterns we are perpetuating are positive and beneficial, this enhances our personal and spiritual growth; conversely, if they are not, the pattern represents a personal block. The blockage could be a relationship, a job, a habit or a way of thinking that we are unable to let go of, so we need to cleanse our chakras of old, nonbeneficial energy to enable them to operate effectively.

A chakra can be described as open, closed or at any of the various stages in between, basically reflecting a person's personality or a reaction to a particular situation. For example, a chakra may be fully open when someone is feeling very happy or safe, or closed when they are feeling ill or threatened, but a blocked chakra may be unable to change its state easily. It may be "stuck" in either an open or closed state, which will affect the general flow of Ki around the physical and energy bodies, and thereby the general state of health of the person. The chakra then needs healing to uncover and remove whatever is blocking it.

You can help to heal a chakra in a number of ways, for instance by working with its element (see the sections on each chakra below); doing physical exercises such as yoga or t'ai chi to relax, open or stimulate the part of the body that it relates to; working with the chakra's associated colors and sounds (see below) or using Reiki to clear blockages in the area and taking steps to change the patterns responsible for the block. However, do be aware that a blockage in one chakra can influence the activity of the chakras above and below it, so for example you may have problems with self-esteem and personal power (third chakra), but this could be influenced by your feelings about sex (second chakra), whereas the real problem may be that you find it difficult to love yourself unconditionally (fourth chakra).

The Seven Major Chakras

Each of the seven chakras is associated with specific parts of the body, and there are further references to this aspect of the chakras' influence in Chapter 5, so in this section I concentrate mainly on the way in which the chakras impact other facets of our lives, and on how to tell whether a chakra is in balance or not.

1. The Base or Root Chakra

The traditional name of this chakra is Muladhara, meaning "root support," and it is located at the perineum, between the genitals and the anus, but is often referred to as being at the base of the spine. It is traditionally associated with the first seven years of life, when our physical growth and mental development are at their height, and its energetic vibrations are linked with the color red, the sound "urrh," the musical note "D," the element earth and the phrase "I have."

This chakra is about how you feel about life and living, and your relationship with your mother and father. Its main influences are to do with survival, physical and material issues, and the will to live, so if your base chakra is in balance your life will generally feel stable, safe and secure, and you will trust in the natural flow of life and the abundance of the Universe. However, when your base chakra is out of balance your life may be governed by a fear of lack, demonstrated by an attachment to money and material possessions and resulting either in hoarding and greed if you are successful in attracting abundance, or poverty and financial worries if you are not. This fear may also manifest as addictions, problems with weight or with food in general, or as a more general fear of the future.

2. The Sacral Chakra

The traditional name of this chakra is Svadhisthana, meaning "one's own place," and it is also sometimes known as the sex center. It is located just below the navel and is traditionally associated with the years between the ages of seven and fourteen, when we are beginning our journey toward sexual maturity. Its energetic vibrations are linked with the color orange, the sound "ooh," the musical note "E," the element water and the phrase "I feel."

144

This chakra is where your body communicates with you about what it needs and what it finds pleasurable, and it is also related to your feelings about having children. One of this chakra's main aspects is therefore our attitude to our own bodies, and to sexuality and sensuality, so a balanced sacral chakra will be shown by an open, healthy and confident attitude to sexual contact, emotional intimacy, desire and sensual pleasures (including enjoyment of food and life in general), expressing creativity (including procreation), and the ability to play and have fun. If your sacral chakra is out of balance, however, this can lead to emotional immaturity, so that instead of forming close, loving relationships you may form imaginary or obsessive attachments, exhibit jealous or manipulative behavior, or have a total fear of intimacy. You may feel unloved and unlovable, leading to feelings of guilt or shame about your own body and ultimately to impotence or frigidity, or to such a lack of care for your own body that you become promiscuous or subconsciously invite sexual abuse.

3. The Solar Plexus Chakra

The traditional name of this chakra is Manipura, meaning "dwelling place of jewels," and it is also sometimes known as the power center. It is located at the solar plexus and is traditionally associated with the years between the ages of fourteen and twenty-one, when we reach physical maturity and begin to "step into our power" and explore our place in the world as adults. Its energetic vibrations are linked with the color yellow, the sound "oh," the musical note "F," the element fire and the phrase "I can."

This chakra is all about your perceptions of power, control and freedom, and being comfortable with yourself, so a balanced solar plexus chakra shows itself in a healthy level of self-respect and self-esteem, allowing you to show consideration for others, without letting their opinions about you affect your sense of your own identity. If you have a balanced solar plexus chakra, your life will reflect a sense of purpose and personal well-being, a flexible, spontaneous approach to people and to life in general, and the ability to stand up for yourself and say no when necessary. With this chakra out of balance, however, you may compensate for a lack of belief in yourself

145

by becoming aggressive, domineering, critical and judgmental, or alternatively you could become very defensive and hypersensitive to criticism and other people's opinions, making you anxious or passive and extremely shy.

4. The Heart Chakra

The traditional name of this chakra is Anahata, meaning "unstruck sound," and it is also sometimes known as the heart center. It is located at the center of the chest and is traditionally associated with the years between the ages of twenty-one and twenty-eight, when we are often exploring our emotions or becoming involved in our first stable sexual/romantic relationships. Its energetic vibrations are linked with the color green, the sound "ah," the musical note "G," the element air and the phrase "I love."

This chakra is about relationships and our perception of love. A heart chakra in balance leads to a compassionate, tolerant, loving and balanced nature, a willingness to help others, and the ability to say "Yes!" to life and to love, which in turn leads to healthy relationships, both with other people and with yourself. If, however, this chakra is out of balance you may develop an unbalanced and unrealistic view of relationships, leading to excessive jealousy, possessiveness or codependency with your partner or children, members of your family or even friends. Sometimes this is demonstrated by an unhealthy need to constantly give and give, and to always "do things for others" without recognizing your own needs, leading to resentment and bitterness. Alternatively, you could become overly fearful of being hurt or rejected, leading to excessive shyness, loneliness and isolation.

5. The Throat Chakra

The traditional name of this chakra is Vishuddha, meaning "purity." It is located at the throat and is traditionally associated with the years between the ages of twenty-eight and thirty-five, a time when we are usually more comfortable with ourselves, and better able to communicate our needs, than we have been in the past. Its energetic vibrations are linked with the color sky blue, the sound "I" (pronounced like eye), the musical note "A," the element spirit and the phrase "I speak."

This chakra is about self-expression, so it is fairly obviously linked with communication on all levels, and when it is in balance you will feel able to communicate freely, clearly, assertively and lovingly, whether in speech, writing, song or other forms of creative or artistic expression. However, it is also about our ability to receive, and our attitude to abundance, as in the phrase "Ask and ye shall receive." So when your throat chakra is out of balance you may find it hard to accept compliments or gifts with good grace, and could lack confidence and find it difficult to express your emotions or opinions. You may speak very quietly or develop a stutter or throat problems, or alternatively, talk incessantly about nothing very important!

6. The Brow Chakra

The traditional name of this chakra is Ajna, meaning "command center," and it is located on the forehead between the eyebrows. It is often called "the third eye," and is generally associated with the years between the ages of thirty-five and forty-two, a time sometimes described as "the midlife crisis," when we begin to reassess our lives and reconsider our priorities and goals for the future. Its energetic vibrations are linked with the color indigo, the sound "Ay," the musical note "B," the element of mind or insight and the phrase "I see."

This is the home of the subconscious and inner vision, and when in balance this chakra allows you to observe and accurately interpret what is going on in your life, so that you can function in a constructive and harmonious way, both personally and with other people. This could mean being very intuitive and responding to spiritual guidance (from your Higher Self), or even having psychic perception such as clairvoyance, but it also means being imaginative or artistic. On the other hand, an imbalance in the brow chakra can lead to problems with physical vision, headaches and difficulty sleeping, as well as to poor memory, an inability to concentrate, and a general lack of understanding or perception about what is going on in your life, even to the stage of being delusional or having hallucinations.

7. The Crown Chakra

The traditional name of this chakra is Sahasrara, meaning "thousand-petalled lotus," and it is located on the top of the head. It is generally associated with the years between the ages of forty-two and forty-nine, when many people begin to seek self-actualization and new meaning in life as their child-rearing responsibilities lessen and they become free to pursue their own vision. Its energetic vibrations are linked with the colors white, gold, purple or violet, the sound "Ee," the musical note top "C," the element light and the phrase "I know."

As the root chakra shows our relationship to the Earth, the crown chakra shows our relationship with heaven, or spirit. A balanced crown chakra brings spiritual awareness, wisdom, inner knowledge and a deep connection to All-That-Is, the consciousness of the Universe, bringing with it a natural desire to develop a spiritual practice such as prayer or meditation—or Reiki! However, an imbalanced crown chakra can lead to you always looking for but never finding the peace and harmony of spiritual connection. This can result in a generally confused state of mind, a tendency to over-intellectualize problems and situations, and either rigid adherence to extreme religious beliefs, or skepticism toward and complete rejection of spiritual matters.

Treating the Chakras with Reiki

When you do a self-treatment with Reiki you are obviously treating your chakras as well as your physical body. If, however, it is your intention to treat a particular chakra, rather than placing your hands directly on your body, it is actually more efficient to hold your hands with your palms facing you, about ten to fifteen centimeters (four to six inches) away from your body, in your aura.

For the crown chakra your hands should be above your head, and for the base chakra your hands should preferably be between your legs, palms facing upward, while for the rest of the chakras your hands would be in front of you (*see illustration below*). The second, third, fourth, fifth and sixth chakras actually emanate from both the front and the back, but it can be rather uncomfortable to try to treat them by holding your hands away from your body with one hand positioned at the back and the other at the front, so position both hands or just one hand in front of you. Your *intention* to treat the chakra will allow the Reiki to flow through both areas.

If you have Second Degree, you will find using the symbols over each chakra very effective. Use the Power Symbol to bring in even more Reiki to help heal and release blockages, and also the Harmony Symbol to help harmonize and balance each chakra.

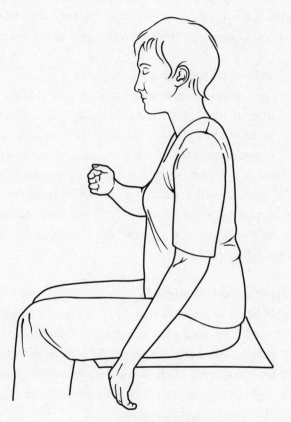

Treating the heart chakra.

You can carry out a full chakra treatment in two ways. The most usual way would be to start at the crown and then work down the energy body, treating the brow, throat, heart, solar plexus, sacral and base chakras, holding each hand position for between two and five minutes. This can be quite tiring, because of course your hands are not supported by your body, so you may find it easier to lie down on a bed or couch or sit in a chair with arms, so that you have somewhere to rest your elbows. (You can bend your head down toward your hands, rather than holding your hands up to your head.)

Alternatively, you can treat all the chakras by starting at the base chakra and working upward. This can have quite an energizing effect but can sometimes leave you feeling a bit "spaced out," so after treating the crown chakra ground the energy by either treating the base chakra again for a minute, or put your feet on the floor and place your hands on your feet, *intending* that Reiki flows through to ground you.

You don't always have to treat all the chakras in this way. You can also use Reiki on an individual chakra, perhaps because you are working on the issues in your life that are linked to that chakra (see the information given on individual chakras on pages 144–148). Hold your hands over the chosen chakra for as long as you feel comfortable— ten to fifteen minutes would be ideal, but you can do this in several five-minute slots, giving your arms a rest for a few minutes in between each slot by placing your hands directly on your body at the location of the chakra. Again, you can use the Power and Harmony Symbols if you have Second Degree.

Linking the Chakras to the Aura

You have probably already realized that since there are seven major chakras and seven layers in your aura, these are connected. It may be helpful to look at the links between them. As I have already mentioned (*see page 40*), each layer of the aura is composed of energy of finer, higher and lighter vibrations, so the first three chakras and the layers of the aura to which they are attached are still associated with the physical dimension, and connected to the body, emotions and mind in a fairly direct way. The heart chakra and the fourth layer of the aura lie between the physical and the spiritual dimensions, acting as a bridge or connecting point, whereas the fifth, sixth and seventh chakras and their associated auric layers are much further away from the physical body, and this is reflected in the fineness of their vibrations and their higher spiritual dimension.

◆ The base chakra is linked to the first layer of the aura, called the **Etheric Body**, which often appears gray-blue in color and is very close to the physical body, perhaps only one or two centimeters (up to about an inch) away, although this distance can expand to five or ten centimeters (two to four inches), especially after you receive a Reiki treatment.

◆ The sacral chakra is linked to the second layer of the aura, called the **Emotional Body**, which varies in depth and can appear to be of any of the seven colors, depending upon the emotions predominant at the time.

◆ Next, the solar plexus chakra is linked to the third auric layer known as the **Mental Body**, which is often seen as a bright golden halo of yellow light radiating around the head and shoulders and is associated with thoughts and mental processes.

◆ The fourth layer of the aura, known as the **Astral Level**, is the link between the physical and the spiritual, and it is connected to the heart chakra. This is associated with our earthly relationships and interactions with other people, creatures and the environment. This layer is sometimes seen as green light, but may also be rosy pink or rainbow colored.

◆ Next is the first of the three higher vibrational fields that have a more spiritual quality. The fifth layer of the aura is known as the **Etheric Template Body**, meaning that it is the energetic "blueprint" for a perfectly healthy Etheric Body, so this is often where blockages or abnormalities can first be detected in the aura. This layer is linked to the throat chakra, and is often fairly transparent and virtually colorless, so that the denser negative energies can be easier to see in it.

◆ The brow chakra, or third eye, is linked to the sixth layer of the aura known as the **Celestial Body**, which is the higher emotional level of the spiritual plane, associated with unconditional (rather than physical) love; it often appears as pastel shades of shimmering colors with a pearlescent quality.

◆ The outer or seventh layer of the aura is called the **Ketheric Template** or **Causal Body**, and it is linked to the crown chakra. This is the mental level of the spiritual plane, associated with bringing our consciousness into oneness with the Source, or All-That-Is. It is the layer that contains both the energetic signatures of your past lives and your current life plan, and it can be seen as various colors, but especially turquoise, gold or lilac.

Using Reiki and Colors to Balance Your Chakras

Color is a powerful force in healing, and you can enhance the effects of Reiki on certain situations by visualizing an appropriate colored light enfolding yourself or a certain part of your body. Clearly, using a color that vibrates to a particular chakra will be especially helpful, so the following visualization uses both Reiki and color to flood each chakra and the whole of your energy field.

◆ Sit in a comfortable position and allow your body to relax. Begin to be aware of your breathing, and follow your breath in and out . . . in and out . . . With each breath you become more and more relaxed. Now imagine and *intend* that you are breathing in Reiki as beautiful bright white light, and see or feel this brilliant white light swirling around, filling your head. With every in-breath the light flows into more of your body. It flows down into your neck, shoulders, and arms, moving right down into your hands until it reaches the very tips of your fingers.

◆ You see or sense the light flowing through your chest and down into your waist and abdomen, and then into your thighs, knees and down into your calves and ankles and into your feet, right to the tips of your toes.

◆ You feel your feet becoming heavier and more solid, and you can feel the connection with the floor beneath you, and then allow the white light of Reiki to flow out of your feet into the earth. Imagine the white light forming roots growing from your feet down into the earth, anchoring you and making you feel very secure.

◆ Now the whole of your body is flooded with the white light of Reiki you can use the Reiki to form a protective barrier around you. Imagine and intend that Reiki is coming out of your hands, and visualize yourself moving your hands over all of your body so that the Reiki forms a cloak of white light surrounding you until each of the seven layers of your aura is filled with the white light of Reiki.

◆ Take your attention back to your body and to your breathing, and imagine and intend that as you breathe in Reiki, its white light begins to slowly change color until you are breathing in warm red light. Allow this red light to flow down and down your body until it reaches your root chakra at your perineum. Feel and intend that the red light is clearing and balancing and opening your base chakra, and then sense it spreading out to fill the lower part of your body, and see it flowing down your legs and into your feet. You can even sense or see it flowing down into the roots of light you have created into the earth.

◆ With your next breath see the Reiki light changing to vibrant orange, and allow this light to flow down your body until it reaches your sacral chakra, near your navel. Feel the orange light clearing and balancing and opening your sacral chakra, and then spreading out to fill your hips, abdomen and all of that part of your body.

◆ Now allow yourself to breathe in Reiki as golden yellow light, and allow this yellow light to flow down your body until it reaches your solar plexus, spreading out to fill that area of your body and clearing, balancing and opening your solar plexus chakra.

◆ Next, the Reiki light changes to a lovely soft green, and as you breathe in this green light it flows down into your chest, where it clears, balances and opens your heart chakra. As it does so it spreads out to fill the whole of your chest, and flows down your arms and into your hands, until even your fingers are filled with this lovely green light.

◆ The Reiki light now changes to a beautiful bright blue, and this blue light fills your throat and neck and you see it swirling around, clearing, balancing and opening your throat chakra.

◆ Your next breath brings in Reiki as a deeper, indigo blue light, and this light flows up into your head, swirling around your brow chakra. You sense it clearing, balancing and opening your third eye.

◆ Finally, you see the Reiki light you are breathing in change to gold or violet or purple—let your intuition choose the color that feels right at this moment—and this light flows up to the top of your head, to your crown chakra. You sense this chakra opening like the petals of a flower, and the Reiki light clears and balances your crown chakra, until the gold or violet or purple light begins to stream out of your crown chakra like a fountain, tinting your whole aura with its delicate colored rays of Reiki light.

◆ Then just enjoy the peace and tranquility of your protected space, and allow any stray thoughts that come into your mind to simply drift across; remain in a relaxed, meditative state for five or ten minutes, or as long as you feel is comfortable. Whenever you are ready, gently allow your eyes to open, stretch your fingers and toes and feel refreshed and alert.

Treating the Chakras with Sound

Another excellent way of clearing and activating your chakras is to use sound. In the sections on each chakra above I have indicated a particular sound and musical note that vibrate in harmony with each chakra. Chanting each sound and note together, for example the sound "Ah" with the musical note "G," between three and seven times, is a very effective and quite energizing activity. It "wakes up" the energy of the chakra and activates the body's Ki energy, and the sound waves help to dislodge blocked energy, allowing it to be released with the voice (although you may need to find somewhere you can do this without disturbing any neighbors—I do it in my car sometimes, while driving!).

Start with the base chakra (the sound is "urrh" and the note is "D"), chanting it three to seven times, and as you repeat it you will probably find that you can hold the note longer and longer. You may get another sound within your head, rather like a single church bell being rung in a slow rhythm. This means you've got the right combination of sound and note. After three to seven repetitions, move on to the sound and note for the sacral chakra, then the solar plexus chakra, and so on. When you have chanted all seven sounds you may feel a little "spaced out," so a quick way of grounding yourself again is to go back to the base chakra sound, chanting "urrh" to the note "D." Doing this once is usually enough, but of course you can continue if you need to.

chapter 8

HEALING YOUR
PHYSICAL SELF

Sadly, despite all the research and technological advances, and despite having the wonderful healing tool of Reiki at your fingertips, there are *no* shortcuts to having a healthy body. You still have to take care of it, and that takes effort. With so much publicity in newspapers, magazines and on television about health and well-being we probably all know by now what we need to do to keep our bodies fit and healthy—but sitting on the sofa reading the articles and watching the programs in order to become better informed is unfortunately not enough! It is probably true that most of us take better care of our cars than we do of our bodies, yet unlike a car, which can be replaced if it wears out, we only get one body per life—it is a one-off opportunity.

If you are interested in having a long and healthy life, it therefore makes sense to look after your body. The rules are relatively simple, but statistics show that unfortunately most of us in the Western world ignore them, leading fairly sedentary lives and stuffing ourselves full of additives, preservatives and drugs like caffeine, nicotine and alcohol. I'm not trying to preach to you—I'm not a perfect example of healthy living myself, although I am trying to be—but just to be sure that we all know what the "rules" are, I give them below.

BODY ESSENTIALS

First and most obviously, we need to breathe, and despite this being such a basic drive, many of us don't breathe well at all. If you watch how a baby breathes, you will see that all of its chest and even its belly move with each inhalation and exhalation, but as we grow up we develop bad breathing habits (as well as possibly taking in cigarette smoke and other pollutants). Many people breathe in quite a fast and shallow way, so they don't use all of their lungs, and over time the reduction in oxygen intake can have a damaging effect on a person's overall health. So a good practice to develop is breathing deeply—so that your belly moves when you breathe—and breathing more slowly, at least some of the time.

Another essential is a nutritionally balanced diet. Put simply, this means that you need to eat at least five portions of vegetables and fruits each day, together with sufficient protein (meat, fish, cheese, eggs, pulses, soya), carbohydrates (rice, bread, potatoes, pasta) and fats (olive oil, soya margarine, butter, fish oils) to give you an adequate amount of vitamins, minerals and fiber. It is also common sense to avoid overeating (or undereating), and to minimize your consumption of sugary foods (cakes, cookies, candy, ice cream), foods high in saturated fats and those that are highly processed (fast food, ready-made fresh or frozen meals, many canned and packaged goods), which tend to contain lots of additives and preservatives.

In addition, you need to drink plenty of water (about two liters/four pints, or eight glasses, of *still* filtered or mineral water each day is the recommendation for adults), and limit your intake of sugary drinks and caffeine (tea, coffee, cola), and of course strictly limit your intake of damaging substances such as tobacco, alcohol and other drugs (although if you are on medication you should continue to take your normal levels of whatever prescription drugs your doctor has authorized).

You also need enough sleep, and usually a bit more in winter than in summer, and some regular physical exercise, preferably three to five times a week. Naturally, the exercise needs to be tailored to your current physical age and condition, so always ask your doctor before you start an exercise regimen—most people need some form of limbering or stretching exercise, such as yoga, as well as aerobic cardiovascular exercise like brisk walking, swimming or cycling.

There are additional factors that have an influence on your potential for optimum health. Where you live and how you live impacts greatly on your health and well-being. Good housing, an unpolluted environment and having caring relationships in our lives are important, as are finding fulfillment in our work or everyday activities, spending time relaxing and having fun, having an opportunity for creative expression and having a sense of purpose. All these are seen as important factors in a healthy lifestyle, and they are often challenged by the kind of stressful, frantically busy lives many of us lead these days.

DETOXING FOR HEALTH

Something that has become quite fashionable in recent years is undertaking a physical "spring-cleaning" by following a gentle detox program. This can have the bonus of helping you to lose excess weight, but its main benefit is that it helps your body to rid itself of toxins, which in turn helps you to look and feel healthier, sleep better, feel calmer and cope more easily with the stresses and strains of modern living.

Your body has its own detoxifiers, namely your liver, kidneys, gut, lymphatic system, skin and lungs, which all get rid of harmful substances and waste products, but they can become overloaded by the sheer volume of toxins they are bombarded with every day. It isn't only the pesticide residues, artificial additives and toxins like alcohol and caffeine in the food and drink we consume that they have to deal with; it's also pollutants in the air such as cigarette smoke and exhaust fumes, and toxins in our homes in detergents and household chemicals, as well as in the environment in the form of mercury and lead.

The basics of a detox are simple. Eat natural, fresh, raw or lightly cooked food, organic wherever possible, cutting out meat, poultry, fish, eggs and dairy products, and limiting certain cereals like wheat. Cut out addictive toxic substances like nicotine, caffeine and alcohol, and cut down on or cut out foods that add to your toxin load, like processed sugars, saturated fats and foods with lots of additives or salt; and drink plenty of water. Did you know that only one in ten adults actually drinks the recommended two liters of water a day, yet drinking just 5 percent less than that can reduce your capacity for concentration and performance by 20 to 30 percent?

You can follow a detox diet for just a few days, or a week, or a month or more, but obviously it can be a good idea to consult your doctor before starting, as detoxing isn't suitable for everyone; for instance, it isn't normally recommended if you're pregnant. The best book I've found is Carol Vorderman's *Detox for Life*—a sensible regimen, with weekly menus, lovely recipes and even a shopping list.

LEARNING TO LOVE YOUR BODY

Unfortunately, few people are satisfied with their bodies, and even fewer people love their bodies. Yet your body is a wonderful, amazing thing; it is through your body that you experience life. But often it is only when something is "wrong" with the body that we learn to appreciate its value. For example, injuring a leg so you cannot walk, or an arm so you cannot wash properly or dress yourself, soon makes you realize how essential those limbs are. Similarly, it is only if you are unfortunate enough to develop impaired sight or hearing that you appreciate how much of life is suddenly "missing" from your experience. One of Dr. Usui's Reiki Principles is "show appreciation" (or "be grateful"), and we need to extend this to appreciating our bodies and to go even further by learning to love them.

Communicating with Your Body

As I described in Chapter 2, our bodies have their own consciousness and wisdom, and they are constantly communicating with us in a loving way—because all the "messages," from illnesses to accidents, are actually expressions of our body's love for us, as it tries to guide us to avoid harm and take the right path. In return, we need to connect to and communicate with our bodies. The following visualization can help you to do that.

◆ Begin by sitting or lying in a comfortable position, and center yourself by breathing deeply and evenly for a few moments. Then let your awareness turn to your body, and imagine and intend that Reiki is flowing into your body, through your crown chakra, and that you are breathing it in through your nose, and that you can see the Reiki as white light.

◆ Watch the light of Reiki surround your whole body, and as you breathe in the Reiki light allow your awareness to follow it through your crown chakra into your head. Allow the Reiki to flow into and around all the bones in your body, and affirm in your mind that you love your skeleton, and that you recognize its value in supporting your body. Let the Reiki flow into all the bones and sockets of the skull, and the bones of your neck and into the collarbones and the shoulders, then down the bones in your arms, wrists, hands and fingers. Now follow the Reiki light down the vertebrae of your spine into your ribs, down further into the bones of the pelvis and then into the bones of your hips, thighs and knees, lower legs, ankles, feet and toes.

◆ Next, allow that Reiki light to flow into your skin, affirming that you love your skin, and you recognize its value as the largest organ of the body, and affirm also that you love your hair and nails and recognize their value. Sense the Reiki flowing into the skin from your toes and toenails all the way up your legs and into your abdomen and chest, and from your bottom up your back to your shoulders. Follow the Reiki down the skin of your arms to the tips of your fingers and fingernails, and then up your neck into your face, scalp and hair.

◆ Now imagine the Reiki light flowing underneath the skin, into all the muscles, tendons, joints and connective tissue, and affirm in your mind that you love your muscles, tendons and joints, and recognize their value in helping you to be supple and flexible. Follow the Reiki light around your body from the muscles in your scalp, face and neck, to the muscles, tendons and joints in your shoulders, arms, hands and fingers, and then into the muscles and tendons in your back, chest and abdomen, and on into the muscles, tendons and joints in your legs and feet.

◆ Next, allow the Reiki to flow into your cardiovascular system, affirming that you love your blood and all its vessels, and acknowledging its vital role in keeping your body alive. Sense the Reiki flowing into your heart, and along all your arteries and veins throughout your whole body, from the heart into your lungs. Pause for a moment, and affirm that you love your lungs and respiratory system, and acknowledge the vital part they play in keeping your body alive. From there follow your blood into your chest and abdomen, down your legs into your feet, and then up to your shoulders and into your arms, neck, face and scalp.

◆ Then let the Reiki light flow into your brain, and affirm that you love your brain and acknowledge its vital role as the command center for your whole body; feel the Reiki flowing into different areas in your brain—the areas for seeing, hearing, speaking, feeling, tasting, touching, smelling, moving; all the areas for communication and for association of ideas; the areas that allow you to coordinate, keep you breathing, digesting, circulating the blood; and the areas that control the rest of your body, the organs, reproductive system and endocrine system. Then let the Reiki flow down your spinal cord and through all the nerves that light up the body, letting it flow into the nerves throughout the arms and hands, the chest and abdomen and back, the legs and feet, and into your neck and head.

◆ Then follow the Reiki light as it flows into your senses, and affirm that you love your senses and recognize their value in letting you interact with the world around you—your eyes so you can see, your ears so you can hear, your nose so you can smell, your mouth so you can taste, your hands, fingers and skin so you can feel and touch.

◆ Next, follow the Reiki light into your mouth and down your throat and into your stomach, intestines and liver, the pancreas, the gallbladder, spleen and bowel, and finally into your kidneys and down into your bladder and out of your body, affirming that you love your digestive system and your excretory system, and recognize their value in helping your body to maintain itself.

♦ Then let the Reiki light flow into your reproductive system, and affirm that you love your reproductive system, including your genitals, and recognize the value of their creative potential and the pleasure they can bring. Sense the Reiki flowing into your genitals and other reproductive organs; from there, let the Reiki light flow into your cells and into your DNA, affirming that you love all of your cells and DNA, and that you recognize the vital part they play in providing your living body.

♦ Now let your awareness move to any part of your body that needs attention right now. Perhaps it isn't functioning properly, or it is tired or in pain, or it might be a part of you that still doesn't feel loved and accepted by you. Place your hands on that part of your body and ask it what it feels, what it needs, or what it wants to tell you; wait for an answer, listening and sensing and giving it your full attention. Words or images or sensations can come from your body's consciousness, so pay attention to them now, noticing what is happening within your body, in your hands, or what thoughts or emotions are going through you. These are your body's messages to you, and the more you do this visualization, the more adept you will become at interpreting the messages, and accessing your body's wisdom.

♦ Now let Reiki flow out of your hands into that part of your body, bringing its peaceful, healing, loving energy to it to gently melt away any pain or tension, and confirm your acceptance, love and appreciation of this part of your body, and of all of your body, gently dissolving any feelings of rejection or lack of self-love. As the Reiki flows into you more and more, sense it bringing fresh energy and vitality to your body, and imagine your body whole, healthy, fit and vibrantly well. See yourself happy and joyful, reveling in any of your favorite activities, such as walking or dancing, with renewed energy and vigor, and see and appreciate how beautiful your body really is.

◆ Spend a little time enjoying this visualization. Then, when you are ready, gradually let yourself become aware of the pressure of your body on the chair or bed and the sounds in the room. Gradually open your eyes and gently stretch your arms and legs until your consciousness has fully returned to the present. Afterward, you may find it useful to write what you experienced in a journal, detailing any impressions or information you received from your body to help with future self-healing.

HEALING AT THE CELLULAR AND DNA LEVELS

Our cells keep replacing themselves daily, and we create virtually a whole new body every year. However, rather like in photocopying, where if you copy a copy many times it isn't as sharp as the original anymore but becomes slightly blurred, the more often a cell replicates, the greater the possibility that any slight imperfections will be magnified. Also, if as some theorists claim, our cells hold our memories and are affected by them, you could say that our pasts are locked into our bodies. But what is really going on is that our consciousness that creates our cells is often locked in the past, in old ways of thinking and feeling and being, and that consciousness keeps re-creating the same old patterns. If, however, we can change the consciousness that creates our cells, then our cells and lives will improve automatically, because health and joy are our natural state. One of the ways of doing this is to use Reiki to heal yourself at a cellular level.

Although at the end of the last visualization we took Reiki into our cells and DNA, this next technique addresses this aspect of our body more specifically and more powerfully. It uses the Power Symbol, but you can try it without: instead of imagining yourself sliding down a symbol, imagine Reiki as a ray of light and slide down that instead.

Healing Your Cells

This is a meditation technique I have devised, using Reiki to heal your cells and DNA.

◆ First, prepare yourself for the meditation by relaxing fully, and becoming centered by breathing slowly and deeply for a few minutes.

◆ When you are ready, imagine yourself standing next to a huge Power Symbol, then visualize both you and the symbol getting smaller and smaller, until you are small enough to fit inside your body. You can imagine yourself inside your head or your chest, whichever you prefer.

◆ Next, take your awareness to the top of the symbol (or a beam of Reiki light) and imagine yourself sitting on it; visualize the spiral below you, rather like a carousel at the fair.

◆ Say the Power Symbol's sacred mantra three times, and intend that the symbol take you into one of your cells—perhaps one that is not currently completely healthy. Now set off—have fun sliding down the symbol or beam of Reiki light until you land (with a plop, of course!) inside one of your cells.

◆ Imagine holding out your hands and letting the Reiki flow from them until the whole cell is filled with Reiki. Intend that the cell be healed, harmonized and balanced by the Reiki until it is totally healthy and glowing with golden light.

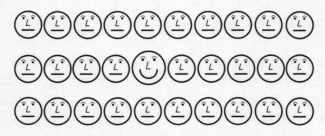

Intend that the cell be healed by the Reiki.

◆ When you have healed one cell, you begin to look around you and you may identify some other cells that are not healthy—perhaps just a few, or even large areas of cells. These may need quite a lot of concentration and determination to fill them with Reiki and golden light, but again, focus on one cell to start with, and allow it to be filled with Reiki and golden light.

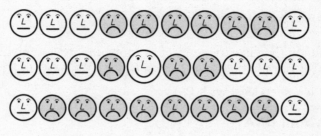

Identify some other cells which are not healthy.

◆ Now imagine that Reiki is flowing out in all directions from that healed cell into the adjoining cells, filling them with golden light until they are also totally healed, harmonized and balanced. As each cell is totally healed, it radiates its perfectly balanced energy and Reiki into its surrounding cells. Slowly but surely the golden glow spreads around your whole body until every cell in your body is filled with Reiki and golden light, glowing with health and in a state of perfect harmony and balance.

◆ When you feel that every cell has been healed, and your body is filled with Reiki energy, allow yourself to slide effortlessly back up the Power Symbol or beam of Reiki light until you are once again sitting on the top. Thank the Reiki for its wonderful healing, and

See every cell filled with Reiki and glowing with health.

165

thank your body for the wonderful job it does in providing a vehicle for you in this life.

◆ Then slowly let the image of yourself sitting on the symbol fade, and let your awareness return to your physical body, to the room in which you are sitting or lying. Open your eyes, and perhaps stretch and shake your hands and feet a little, to bring your consciousness fully back into the present.

◆ You might then like to spend a few more minutes just giving yourself Reiki and enjoying the relaxed and glowing feeling of being filled at a deep level with Reiki.

Healing Your DNA

You can follow exactly the same procedure as the meditation above, but this time slide down the Power Symbol (or a beam of Reiki light) into your DNA. See its intertwining strands, and ask and *intend* that Reiki flows into your DNA, healing and transforming your DNA until it gives you the optimum healthy genetic coding you need to fulfill your true potential in this life. Remember to thank the Reiki and your body afterward, as before. Below is a diagram of DNA, in case you find it difficult to imagine what it looks like.

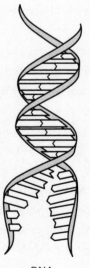

DNA.

THE EFFECTS OF REIKI ON YOUR BODY

When you use Reiki on yourself, how does it actually affect the body? Well, because Reiki is an energy of a much higher vibration than the denser, physical energy of which your body is comprised, it can permeate all areas of the body, nourishing them with an even higher vibration than your own life force, or Ki. This supports and accelerates your body's own natural ability to heal itself by bringing it into balance.

As an example of how this operates, one of my students worked in an intensive care unit and when she touched patients Reiki would almost always flow through her into them (because their Higher Selves knew they needed Reiki, they would draw it). She would almost immediately see the reactions in their bodies, because they were attached to various monitoring machines. If their blood pressure was too high, it would begin to go down; if it was too low, it would begin to go up. If their heart rate or respiration was too fast, it would begin to slow down, or if it was too slow, it would speed up. To give another example: I sent a number of distant Reiki treatments over a week to a patient who had had a triple bypass heart operation, and the medical staff were amazed at the rate at which the wound was healing—so rapidly, in fact, that when they came to remove the tubes, they had to cut them away.

Reiki can also help to alleviate pain and relieve other symptoms. Such symptoms are signs that there is a problem, blockage or imbalance in the body; Reiki flows into the blockage and its high vibrational energy dissolves and dissipates the denser energies of the blockage. This is also how Reiki helps to cleanse the body of poisons and toxins—these also affect the body's chemical balance, and Reiki balances and harmonizes the denser energies in the body, allowing them to be eliminated by the normal excretory system, or to be released through the energy body. The eventual result is that Reiki promotes a sense of wholeness, a state of positive wellness and an overall feeling of well-being. It also works with your physical consciousness, or body wisdom, to help you develop a greater awareness of your body's real needs, for example encouraging a realization that you need a better diet, or more exercise or a better sleep pattern.

It is, however, important to realize that this does not mean that Reiki always effects a cure. It will almost always have some beneficial effect at the physical level, but remember that it always works for your highest and greatest good, which actually may not be served by eliminating a physical illness. There may be deeper, subconscious reasons for continuing to have an illness or disease, based on your mental, emotional or spiritual needs, such as requiring the time off work to give you a chance to review your life and your priorities—the ailment could be a "wake-up call."

REIKI HAND POSITIONS FOR GENERAL ILLNESS

Dr. Usui had several techniques that employed particular hand positions for dealing with illness. One of them, *Genetsu-ho*, was apparently used for many diseases, but was particularly useful for treating anything involving fever or inflammation. In Japanese *Ge* means to bring down, *Netsu* means fever and *Ho* means treatment, method or way.

1. Sit or lie down comfortably, then place one or both hands on your forehead for several minutes and *intend* that Reiki should flow for your greatest and highest good.

2. Move your hands to your temples and let Reiki flow for several minutes.

3. Place your hands at the back of your head, letting Reiki flow for several minutes.

4. Place one hand at the back of your neck and the other on your throat for several minutes.

5. Place one (or both) hands on your crown for a few minutes.

6. Place one hand on your stomach (solar plexus area) and the other hand over your intestines (sacral area) for several minutes.

7. Remove your hands from your body, place them in the *Gassho* position, and give thanks for the Reiki, ending with a bow of respect.

Another similar technique called *Byogen Chiryo* was apparently used by Dr. Usui to help to get to the root of a physical problem, regardless of where in the body the symptoms appeared. Sometimes when using this technique you will receive intuition about the physical and metaphysical causes behind the illness or disease. *Byo* means disease in Japanese, *Gen* means origin or root, and *Chiryo* means medical treatment.

1. Sit or lie down comfortably. Place one hand behind your neck and the other in front of your throat, and let Reiki flow for your greatest and highest good for about five minutes, or longer if you feel this is necessary.

2. Place one (or both) hands on your crown, letting Reiki flow for five minutes or more.

3. Place one hand on your stomach (solar plexus area) and the other over your intestines (sacral area), again holding your hands there for five minutes or more.

4. Remove your hands from your body, place them in the *Gassho* position and give thanks for the Reiki, ending with a bow of respect.

SELF-HEALING FOR SERIOUS ILLNESS

I have already mentioned in an earlier chapter that self-healing can take time, commitment, determination and perseverance, but they are even more important in the case of chronic or life-threatening illnesses. If you have a really serious illness, or have suffered an accident leading to multiple injuries, then there are two main possibilities: it could be your chosen way to leave your physical body (although chosen at the level of your Higher Self, not your conscious self), or it could be your body's final desperate attempt to get your attention—a last "cry for help." Whichever of these situations it is, as well as gaining insight into the causative levels of your illness—for chronic, severe or life-threatening illnesses are rarely the result of a single cause—you have another important lesson to learn: to make *yourself* your number one priority. This means giving yourself the time it takes—however much time that is—to carry out your self-healing, perhaps on a 24/7 basis for many weeks, months or even years. That takes a great deal of commitment, patience and courage—courage to say no to other people—even those you care deeply about—and no to yourself by letting go of many other commitments, including work, church, golf club, playgroup committee, and so on, even if they have always meant a lot to you. In her book *The Invitation*, Oriah Mountain Dreamer talks about the courage it takes to draw back from looking after other people to concentrate on looking after yourself, but if you are serious about self-healing and your physical body is demonstrating some form of serious illness, then that is what it takes. There are many well-known people involved in self-healing, such as Louise L. Hay and Brandon Bays, who managed to heal themselves of very serious conditions like cancer, but for them it took single-minded determination and virtually twenty-four-hours-a-day effort to achieve this. This is the level of dedication you need for your self-healing of any serious illness, too, and not just at the beginning, but through all the stages, including what could be a lengthy period of recuperation.

Can you imagine changing your whole lifestyle, including sleeping much more and eating the healthiest possible diet to give your body the best chance to heal itself? Treating yourself with Reiki for up to twelve hours or even more each day? Doing a visualization for ten minutes every hour where you see yourself whole and healthy? Listening to self-help tapes or CDs for several hours a day? Nurturing yourself by having several aromatherapy massages each week? Taking homeopathic treatments, such as Bach Flower Remedies, maybe having acupuncture, counseling, NLP sessions, and so on, and so on—in fact, actively pursuing anything and everything that might help? And can you envisage asking someone to look after *you* for a change?

It sounds tough, doesn't it? It also sounds like a huge amount of effort, and it probably goes against your normal instincts to be so self-absorbed. But it isn't selfish, because if your life is important to you and to the people who love you, and that's what it takes, then that's what you have to do. Thinking positively, believing that returning to full health is a possibility, plays its part, too. It's no good putting in all that effort if you're convinced it's going to fail anyway, because your negative attitude will actively be working against your self-healing, making it much less effective. Reiki and many other therapies can help, but in the end it is still you and your body, in conjunction with your Higher Self, that does the healing.

Work through the self-healing stages: acknowledge that you are ill and you need help; accept that for the time being your illness is your number one priority; seek awareness of the causative levels; and take as active a part in your self-healing as you can. Believe in the best possible outcome and it can become a reality, but if for some reason, despite all the self-healing you do, whatever disease you have is still not cured, the depth of healing generated by so much inner work being done on all levels will allow you to make your transition, when it comes, with peace and dignity, and with the knowledge for yourself and your family and friends that you did all you could.

CELEBRATING YOUR PHYSICAL LIFE

Life is precious, and accepting and learning to love your body is an important part of celebrating your physical life, whatever physical shape you are in, or whatever illnesses, impairments or disabilities you may have. You can still find ways of enjoying your body and loving it. For example, you might strengthen your body by learning yoga, t'ai chi or chi kung, or by taking up some form of exercise like swimming or cycling. You could perhaps join up with friends and go walking or sailing, because spending time in nature is so uplifting; even if you can only get as far as your garden or a local park to experience some fresh air and practice your deep breathing, it will still help you to feel better.

Another way of loving your body is to treat it to some relaxation. That could include something as simple as a luxuriously scented bubble bath, or some time spent listening to beautiful music, or you could go for an aromatherapy massage, or some shiatsu or a reflexology treatment. You could also go to a practitioner for a Reiki treatment, even if you self-treat every day. I make sure I go once a month, because you can reach an even deeper level of relaxation and "letting go" when being treated by someone else.

The important thing is to learn to enjoy life—to live each day as if it was your last. If you really had only one day to live, you wouldn't waste it on regrets, being bad-tempered or moaning about being mistreated, by, would you? You'd want to savor life. To "wake up and smell the coffee," as the saying goes. Every sensation would be precious, from the sight of a partner's smile to the sound of a child's laugh, from the sweet smell of fresh air to the taste of a lovingly prepared meal. That's what life's all about, really. So celebrate it!

Of course, it makes sense to take a good look at your life to see if it is helping or hindering you in achieving optimum holistic health. Are you eating a really healthy diet, or snatching fast food on the run to your next meeting? Are your major relationships—with partners, children, siblings, parents and close friends—healthy and loving or stressful and tense? Are you happy with whatever work you do, whether it is in external employment or in the home, or do you really long to do something else? Do you have time to indulge in hobbies and interests that add to your life, or are you always working or rushing around making everyone else's lives easier? Have you achieved some of your dreams and goals and do you expect to achieve even more, or have you given up the unequal struggle and settled for whatever you can get? Do you think life is wonderful, fun and a joy, or do you find it all too much of an effort, and cannot think why you bother?

Take some time to think about these questions, because being happy with your life has tremendous benefits for your physical health, and conversely of course, being unhappy can be detrimental to your health. In the next few chapters we will be looking at healing your emotional, mental and spiritual self, so you may find some ideas that will help you to identify areas in your life that you need to work on, and methods to help you do so.

chapter 9

HEALING YOUR
EMOTIONAL SELF

We tend to use the words "feelings" and "emotions" interchangeably, but there are differences between them. Feelings are physical sensations, such as hunger, pain, tiredness or more positive feelings such as feeling fit and well, so at some level we are all experiencing feelings most of the time. They are simple reactions to what is happening in the moment, and pure feelings have no emotional content. They simply "are."

Emotions, however, result when feelings are filtered through our beliefs, when we develop judgments about what we should, or should not, be feeling. For example, pain is an unpleasant physical sensation, and not unnaturally we want to get rid of pain and get back to feeling well again. However, we have choices about how we react to pain. We could simply accept it, for example by thinking "I've got a headache," and taking an aspirin (or give ourselves Reiki!) to get rid of it. But if we believe our headache is the result of having to work long hours for an uncaring employer, or is because we have noisy neighbors, we might feel angry about it; or if we believe the headache could be a symptom of something more serious, we might feel afraid. These are emotional responses rather than physical feelings.

We also experience psychological feelings, and these too can just be acknowledged without necessarily having an emotional content. Take a simple example. You are walking behind someone toward a door and instead of holding the door open to let you through as well, they let it slam shut in front of you. You might feel surprised, but your reaction could be to just accept what has happened, open the door again and walk through. If, however, you judge the other person's action as being a rejection of you, challenging your sense of personal worth, or if you believe that it is rude to act like that, then you could imbue the event with an emotion. You might feel hurt, sad, angry or disgusted, and you might also believe that such an emotion has been caused by that person or that event.

Emotions, however, are not caused by outer events. Emotions are an internal reaction to an external event, and that is very different. If someone sticks a pin into you and it hurts, that's an external event causing a feeling—pain. But if someone sticks a pin into you and you get angry about it, or scared that they might do it again, or emotionally hurt because you can't understand why they would do such a thing, then those emotions are internal reactions. They represent a choice you have made. We choose what emotion to feel. Always. So emotions aren't automatic reactions to situations or events; they form a part of our complex responses to life—our personalities—which are based on our life experiences so far. This is why different people react in diverse ways to the same situations.

EMOTIONAL PROGRAMMING

You have been receiving emotional programming since you were a small child, and in your early years this would have been from your parents and siblings, and from teachers and friends. However, in the modern world this programming can also come from television and films, because these reflect images of emotions to which we are susceptible, especially when we're young. Think of the huge range of emotions, from intolerable grief to overwhelming happiness, sexual desire to violent anger, demonstrated in any of the soap operas on television, for example. It is this emotional programming that is one of the foundations for our belief system, which we integrate into our subconscious, and which then provides us with our patterns of behavior and our habitual emotional responses.

Psychological research has shown that if either or both of your parents showed little emotion, laughing or crying infrequently, and rarely or never hugging or holding you, then you are likely to grow up suppressing your emotions, because you believe that is the way to be. Alternatively, you may have been exposed to a parent who was overly emotional—who cried easily, or lost their temper regularly—so this would be the "norm" to you, and you would be likely to follow in their footsteps.

We all learn by example, and what we learn is eventually absorbed into our own personalities, so that the pattern continues from one generation to another. Of course, we have other choices. Sometimes people react against their programming, and if their childhood was miserable because of harsh or restrictive and unloving parents, they will behave in the opposite way when they are adults, becoming loving, tolerant and demonstrative. But that only goes to show that we choose our emotions and the way we express them. Just because we have formed a subconscious habit of reacting to certain situations in a certain way doesn't mean we have to continue the habit forever. We can change our reactions.

CARRYING OUT EMOTIONAL HEALING

The first thing I need to say is don't be ashamed of your feelings or emotions. They are valid parts of you as you are at this moment, and even if you do want to change it is OK to be who you are and where you are right now. To reject and suppress your feelings and emotions would cause you even more problems, so remember the first step to self-healing (*see page 29*), and start by acknowledging how you feel and realizing that the way you feel is a lot to do with your upbringing and the many experiences you have had in your life so far. Perhaps I should add that you shouldn't blame your parents, siblings, teachers and friends for behaving the way they did, because everyone does the best they can, with the knowledge and experience they have. We are all products of our life experiences, and when we learn new and better ways of behaving and dealing with things, we usually adopt those new ways. But you can't do what you don't know!

No matter how hard parents, teachers or other significant people in our lives try, as children we inevitably experience some degree of emotional hurt, neglect or feelings of rejection or abandonment, and because we're so vulnerable as children we can be deeply wounded by these experiences. We can carry these feelings inside us into adulthood and even throughout our lives—or at least until we do some emotional healing work. Underneath our emotions lie our basic needs for love, acceptance, security and self-esteem, and when we work on our emotional healing, we are learning to give to ourselves what we didn't get as small children.

A good place to start is to look back to your childhood and to your relationships with your parents, grandparents, brothers and sisters, and perhaps your wider family—aunts, uncles and cousins. Getting out the family photo albums can help to let some memories rise to the surface. Do you remember your parents praising you a lot, or were they perhaps quite critical? Did your grandparents spoil you? Did you have a favorite aunt or uncle, and if so, why?

Looking back and analyzing what happened to you can help you to realize why you are the person you are today. And of course, you will have grown through some things already—you are a unique individual, so you will have rejected some of your earlier programming in order to develop your own way of being. For instance, you may have been jealous of a younger brother because you thought he was cleverer than you, or hated an older sister because she was prettier than you. Once you all became adults those old emotions will hopefully have passed into history along with the teddy bear or tricycle you fought over!

Whatever childhood experiences you had in the past need to be acknowledged, but they don't need to continue influencing your life. You can move on to the next stage in the healing process—acceptance. What happened, happened, and you are what you are. Some of the people who were close to you when you were a child may even have died or moved away, yet you may still be carrying with you some of the emotional "baggage" that you collected because of something they said or did.

You may have fears about security that have made you very materialistic; a lack of self-esteem that is holding you back in your career; a love life that's littered with failed relationships because no matter how much a lover protests, you don't believe, deep down, that you're lovable. Whatever stage you are at, it is possible to change, to heal the past, to let go of emotional baggage and move on, to forgive the people who influenced you—and to forgive yourself, because sometimes we can feel guilty for letting ourselves be influenced in this way.

Be willing to take steps slowly. Doing emotional healing can be tough and upsetting as you move through the layers of laid-down pain. But think of it this way. If you had twenty-five kilos (about 55 pounds) in excess layers of fat that you wanted to get rid of, it would take time and effort, wouldn't it? You'd have to keep to a sensible diet and do some physical exercise, and sometimes you'd feel daunted by the prospect of keeping up a strict regimen for months on end—but once you were fit and trim you would look back and realize it had all been worth it. Well, emotional healing can be much the same. It will take time and effort, but you will eventually feel so much better and happier, even if sometimes during the healing process you hit really low points.

EMOTION IS EITHER LOVE OR FEAR

There is a popular concept that everything that is not love is fear, and that therefore all unwanted or negative emotions are based on fear. But fear of what? Fear of rejection, pain, abandonment, making a fool of oneself, lack (for instance not enough money/food to live on) and even fear of death are just some of the baseline fears leading to emotions such as jealousy, possessiveness, greed, nervousness, depression, sadness, anger, and so on. So the next stage of the healing process involves developing an awareness of what is at the root of an emotion. What is it you are afraid of?

This can be a pretty scary question to ask yourself. This is because fear is an emotion that most of us try hard to get rid of, or at least to bury or hide, which is why we find so many other names for the emotion of fear. But fear can serve a useful purpose. It warns us that something may be difficult or dangerous so that we will pay attention, evaluate the situation and choose some appropriate action. As an example, let's look at the fear of rejection. That can make us very shy or self-effacing, so we will avoid putting ourselves in situations where we might be rejected. This in turn stops us from going to a party where we might meet someone new, or applying for a job that might challenge us too much, or asking someone for a date because they might say no.

But the baseline issues behind all of these fears are a lack of self-esteem, a lack of acceptance of ourselves as we are and not being able to love ourselves. If we love ourselves, the opinions of other people become far less important, and we can take risks because whatever the result it won't hurt us emotionally.

If we love ourselves we can ask someone for a date because we know they might say yes, but if they say no we won't take it as a personal insult. It just means they don't want to go out with us—and that's fine. Someone else will. We will apply for a job that seems interesting and challenging, and if we don't get it, that's OK. Someone else may have been more suited to it on the day, but that doesn't mean there's anything wrong with us. Another chance will come along, and next time we might be successful. See what I mean? If we develop more and more love for ourselves, we can let go of more and more fears. It's a simple equation, but it works!

Of course, I'm not talking about the kind of self-love that results in someone being egocentric, bigheaded, vain and self-absorbed. By loving yourself I mean having tolerance, compassion and self-respect for yourself, and caring for yourself—an understanding that whatever "faults" you may have, actually at a deep level you are an OK person; that at this moment in time, with the knowledge and understanding you have, you are perfect exactly the way you are. That doesn't mean you can't strive to become even better. Neither does it mean that you don't need to continually extend your insight and self-awareness, your personal growth and spiritual development. It just means that right here, right now, you're OK. (I would recommend the book *I'm OK, You're OK*, by Thomas A. Harris, M.D., as a very good starting point for understanding this issue.)

USING REIKI FOR EMOTIONAL HEALING

Once you've developed an awareness of the causative factors behind your emotions, the next stage in the healing process is action. One way of carrying out emotional healing is to use Reiki. There are advantages to being able to use the Reiki symbols for this, but you can simply let the Reiki flow and it will do its job, although it may take just a little longer.

1. First, decide which emotions you want to work on. (You can work on more than one emotion at a time, but it is best to link similar types of emotion together.) You might choose to deal with one or more of the following: fear, nervousness, depression, anger, sadness, grief, impatience, anxiety or any other emotion that you feel needs healing.

2. Decide where you generally feel these emotions. For example, anger, fear or problems with self-esteem are often felt in the solar plexus; loneliness, grief or rejection in the heart chakra; money or job worries in the base chakra; jealousy about sexual relationships in the sacral chakra, and so on. (Look back at the hand positions for self-treatment in Chapter 5, or the details about the chakras in Chapter 7, for more information.)

3. If you have Second Degree, draw or imagine a large Harmony Symbol and Power Symbol over what seems to be the most appropriate chakra (if you're not sure which one it should be, draw the symbol over your crown chakra). Visualize the symbol expanding until it encompasses the whole of you, say its mantra three times, and ask and *intend* that it brings its gentle, healing, peaceful and restorative energy to fill your physical and energy bodies, to bring greater harmony and balance to your life, and to heal your feelings of . . . (name whatever emotion(s) you want to work on).

4. If you don't have Second Degree, place both your hands over the appropriate chakra, and imagine and *intend* that Reiki is flowing

out of your hands, and ask and *intend* that Reiki heals, harmonizes and balances your physical and energy bodies, to bring greater harmony and balance to your life, and to heal your feelings of . . . (name the emotion(s) you want to work on).

5. Let yourself stay in a meditative state, giving yourself Reiki, and imagine being surrounded and encompassed by Reiki for at least five minutes, but preferably for about fifteen minutes, until you feel much calmer and more content. Then either take your hands away and place them in the *Gassho* (prayer) position, giving thanks to Reiki with a little bow, or if you have Second Degree, draw a Power Symbol to seal in the peaceful energies, saying its mantra three times, and then *Gassho* and give thanks.

6. Finally, clap your hands or shake them vigorously to break the energy connections.

7. Repeat this exercise on a daily basis, working with one or more emotions until you sense that they have changed, and feel less strong or less troublesome. A good check for this is to think of some situation that would normally trigger the type of emotion you are working on, let yourself really imagine it as vividly as possible and see if you get any reaction in the appropriate chakra or part of your body. If you don't, then at least some healing has occurred—but of course you can always repeat the process any time those emotions resurface (if they ever do).

DEALING WITH NEGATIVE EMOTIONS

Another way of working on emotional healing is to express and let go of negative emotions. Repressed feelings become blocked energy, which can then become emotional and physical ailments, but allowing ourselves to express feelings can create free-flowing energy and thereby create emotional and physical health and well-being.

Negative emotions become trapped when we refuse to let them out, either because we are too polite or too frightened to express them verbally, or because we suppress our feelings out of habit. But releasing emotion can be much easier than you think. It just needs to be made external, rather than remaining internal. This can be done through speech, writing, art, physical action, singing, chanting, drumming, pillow beating, and so on.

What you do *not* need to do is to say nasty or angry things directly *to* any person, because the aim is to release and heal your emotions, not dump them on someone else. There is therefore no need to shout verbal abuse at someone with whom you feel angry or upset, although you can describe your feelings about a person and their actions to someone else, if that is what helps to make you feel better. We probably all know the value of having a good "moan" to someone about our partner, or boss or an unhelpful authority figure!

Writing things down can be good therapy, so writing a letter to someone, telling them exactly how you feel (but *not* mailing it!) helps to release your negative emotions, allowing you to become calmer and better able to look at the situation from a different perspective. An alternative is to write a poem about the situation, or some song lyrics or a short story (changing the names and some other details, of course). Writing a story is particularly good, because you can work through all the emotions with each character, and the dialogue can include all the things you wish you'd said—and of course you can invent the outcome you want. If you feel you need to speak or shout or scream the emotions out, then go somewhere where you cannot be heard by anyone else, or turn on some loud music, for example.

Painting can be a wonderful release, too, and you don't even need to be particularly artistic to use this method. Just sloshing some paint on a piece of paper—especially lots of red, orange and yellow if you're feeling angry—can be fun as well as therapeutic. Physical activity—running, punching the air, kicking the air, lifting weights or swimming fast (if you are fit enough) are all good ways to get rid of pent-up emotion. Singing loudly, beating a drum, playing a musical instrument (loudly) or bashing a pillow with your fists are also good ways of letting out feelings, but again, most of those might need you to be somewhere out of the way of other people, or they may have to be disguised with other sounds, such as singing in the shower. Do experiment—finding a safe way of releasing your emotions, without harming anyone or damaging anything, will allow you to feel so much better.

EMOTIONAL HEALING FOR THE PAST

This next technique ideally needs the symbols taught at Second Degree to enable you to send Reiki into the past so that it can heal past events or hurts. Doing this will not physically alter what has happened—although it will have an impact energetically—but it can allow healing and forgiveness to permeate that time, and this will gently alter the way you feel about it now. This is therefore a good technique to use to "let go" of any regrets or anger you might feel about how you were treated as a child. For example, if you had a difficult or traumatic experience in the past with one or more of your relatives, and you know the approximate date when this happened, you can use the Distant (Connection) Symbol to send Reiki back to that time to heal the trauma.

It often helps if you incorporate a photograph of yourself close to the time of the event in question into this technique. If, however, you don't know the date of the event, or don't have a photo, the technique will still work if you just name the problem and ask that Reiki go to the cause and heal it.

1. Write down a brief description of the situation and include the rough timing (for example a broken relationship with X when you were twenty years old). Draw or imagine the Distant Symbol over the paper (and photograph of you at that age, if you have one), and silently say its sacred mantra three times, sensing it connecting the you of today with the you of that time.

2. Draw or imagine the Harmony Symbol over the paper/photo and repeat the mantra three times, sensing its healing flowing to the

hurt and upset, and to the root cause and the lessons you were meant to learn from the event.

3. Draw or imagine the Power Symbol over the paper/photo and repeat the mantra three times, sensing a strong flow of Reiki moving into that time.

4. Allow the Reiki to flow for ten to fifteen minutes, or longer if it feels appropriate. Then draw the Power Symbol over the paper/photo and repeat the mantra three times, *intending* that the healing be sealed in for the greatest and highest good. Clap your hands to break the connection, and let go of that event in your thoughts.

If you don't have Second Degree, try holding the photo or piece of paper with the details of the past event in your hands, and ask Reiki to flow into it. This may take a bit longer than the above technique, and you may have to do it a number of times, but the Reiki can still have a beneficial effect—the symbols just allow it to happen faster.

If in the days following this activity you get a sense that the healing is not complete—perhaps you've dreamed about the event, or it has entered your thoughts quite a few times, unexpectedly—then repeat the above instructions, again sending Reiki to the same situation. You can do this as many times as necessary, but once is often enough. Sometimes it is just the way you've worded the situation that is preventing the healing from being completed—you might, for example, be trying to send the Reiki to the other person involved, which would be ethically incorrect.

You can only have responsibility for your own self-healing, but by healing your own reactions to and thoughts about a particular time or event, that healing automatically flows outward, rather like the ripples made by a pebble thrown into a pond. It gradually permeates through the energetic signature of the whole situation, allowing any other people involved to receive whatever healing their Higher Selves deem to be necessary.

Healing your own part in an event can therefore have some extra-ordinary effects—I have known family members who haven't spoken to each other for years because of a family feud to suddenly get in touch again when students of mine have sent Reiki to the original situation. Healing their *own* feelings about it helped others to recognize this on a subconscious, energetic level, so that they too could heal their own part in it.

HEALING YOUR CURRENT RELATIONSHIPS

I have discussed relationships from your past and how these influence your emotions, but what about relationships you have now? You may have tension in your family, or difficult relationships with a partner or ex-partner, with your parents or children, or with a friend or acquaintance. Perhaps there's scope for healing there, too. See if there are any patterns emerging. For example, if you had a very domineering father or brother, have other men in your life been of a similar type? If your mother was very possessive and clingy, do you attract women friends or partners like that, or do you go for the complete opposite? (This isn't an attempt to psychoanalyze yourself, just a way to raise your awareness a little.)

Whatever problems you are having, from strained relationships with your partner or family, to difficulties with colleagues at work, you can use Reiki to help to permeate the situation with healing. Below you will find a couple of exercises that you can repeat as often as necessary—even on a daily basis—until the relationship shows signs of developing greater harmony or it changes in some other way.

Of course, Reiki works for your highest and greatest good, and we don't always know what that is, even if we think we do. You may, for instance, wish Reiki to heal and harmonize your relationship with your wife, husband or partner, so that whatever problems you are experiencing will melt away and you can "get back to normal." However, your greatest good (and that of your partner) may be better served in the long term by the relationship breaking up, in which case Reiki won't just paper over the cracks. Instead, it may raise your awareness of why your relationship isn't working so that you can let it go with love, rather than clinging on out of habit. In other words, there is no point in having specific expectations of what Reiki will do—it will just do what it needs to do for your highest and greatest good.

Part I—Writing Down the Situation

1. Sit quietly in a comfortable position and center yourself, allowing your breathing to settle into a deep, slow rhythm.

2. Think about the problem you want to work on, and write down the details on a piece of paper. Examples could be "Allow Reiki to flow into the situation of my relationship with my father, for the highest and greatest good," or "Let Reiki flow into the situation of the family tension over my divorce, for the highest and greatest good."

3. Hold the paper between your hands, and allow Reiki to flow into it for five or ten minutes. If you have Second Degree you can also draw the Harmony Symbol and the Power Symbol over the paper, saying their sacred names three times.

4. After five or ten minutes, place the piece of paper somewhere safe so that you can repeat the process again tomorrow. It can be a good idea to place it under a crystal that you have charged with Reiki (*see page 240*) so that the situation continues to receive the gentle harmonizing energy of Reiki throughout the day. Then *Gassho*, give thanks to Reiki and get on with your day.

Part II—Visualizing the Situation

1. Sit quietly in a comfortable position and center yourself, allowing your breathing to settle into a deep, slow rhythm.

2. Think about which relationship you want to work on, for example that between you and your partner, or you and a work colleague (or several colleagues).

3. Let yourself visualize the people involved as clearly as possible—but bear in mind that you're not aiming for Technicolor Panavision Widescreen! Simply remembering what they, and you, look like is all that is required.

4. Imagine the pairs or groups of people you want to work on all together, perhaps sitting on a sofa or around a table.

5. Hold your hands out at a comfortable distance in front of you, about thirty centimeters (twelve inches) apart, as if they are encompassing the image, and allow Reiki to flow, asking and *intending* that it bring its healing energy to the situation between you and the other person(s). Hold that image for about five minutes—or longer, if you wish. You can turn it into an imaginary "film" if you want, seeing the people involved talking together, getting on better, maybe laughing and perhaps ending with a hug.

6. If you have Second Degree, you can also draw the Distant Symbol to connect to the group, the Harmony Symbol to bring peace and harmony to the situation, and the Power Symbol to supply healing energy. Repeat their mantras three times, and give a brief description of the group once (for example, my wife and I; or Bob, Linda, Paul and myself at work). Then imagine the Harmony Symbol hovering above the group, and watch it gently descend until it encompasses the whole group. *Intend* that it bring its peaceful, harmonious energies to the group, for the greatest and highest good, and hold this image for about five minutes. As suggested above, you can turn this into a moving visualization, seeing the people involved getting on better, and ending with a handshake or a hug or kiss, as appropriate. Then draw the Power Symbol, say its mantra three times, and *intend* that the healing is complete.

7. Finally, clap your hands or shake them vigorously to break the connection. Sit quietly for a few more minutes, hands in the

Gassho position, giving thanks to the Reiki and bringing yourself back to a centered and calm state. (Sometimes doing this exercise can make you feel very emotional, and if so, that's fine—just let the tears flow, as this is a good form of release, and it shows that the healing has already begun.)

Of course, you cannot determine the outcome of this exercise, because the Reiki will always be acting for your highest and greatest good, but generally you will find that there will be some improvement, as the people involved will be aware, on an energetic level (and through their Soul/Higher Self), that you are trying to create greater harmony for the good of you all.

You can also do this exercise to help you with other types of contact, such as meetings or interviews. In those cases do the same as above, but perhaps imagine the appropriate group of people sitting around a table. If you don't know all their names, or what they look like, it doesn't matter: just specify "all the people at my interview," or "all the people at the Council meeting," or whatever the case may be. If you have Second Degree you can use the Distant Symbol and specify the time of the meeting or interview; when you hold the image of the group, you can perhaps "see" the meeting ending with everyone smiling and shaking hands.

LETTING GO OF NEGATIVE RELATIONSHIPS

Even though we may have moved miles away from our family, or have left a relationship that went sour, energetically we may still be connected. It can be difficult to stop thinking about past hurts that have led to the breakdown of relationships with members of our families or former partners, but those thoughts and emotions can keep us tethered, even though we might think we have broken free.

Each important person in our lives forms an energetic connection to us, and these connections can be seen by some psychic people as cords or strands, usually joining from the heart or solar plexus chakras

187

of both people, although other chakras may also be involved. These cords can be present regardless of the distance between them. Here is a simple visualization to help you to disconnect from any unhealthy or negative relationship.

1. First, allow yourself to become centered by breathing deeply and evenly, then protect yourself with Reiki, either by allowing Reiki to flow out of your hands and imagining it filling a bubble of light around you, or by drawing the Power Symbol in front, behind and on each side of you and *intending* that the Reiki protect you.

2. Decide which relationship you wish to detach from, and imagine the other person involved climbing into the basket beneath a hot-air balloon that is tethered to the ground.

3. Ask your Higher Self to reveal to you any cords or strands that are connecting you to this person, and as your inner vision becomes clearer you may be amazed at how many there are, and how thick some of them are.

4. Now imagine that someone is beginning to loosen the ropes that are holding the basket on the ground, and that the hot-air balloon is beginning to lift up into the air. Be aware of the cords or strands between you and the other person stretching up as the basket lifts higher.

5. Imagine that you have in your hands a pair of golden scissors, and begin to cut the cords one by one. Some of them may be very resistant, but persevere, and if the golden scissors don't seem to be strong enough, then a golden knife or ax or hacksaw will be available, and you can use that instead.

6. Gradually, as each of the cords is severed, imagine that the cords withdraw back into each person's chakras, and intend that Reiki flows to heal the wound, both in your own energy body and in the other person's energy body.

7. When all of the cords have been cut (some of them may try to reattach themselves, so you may have to cut them again) imagine the hot-air balloon flying higher and higher up into the sky. *Intend* and affirm that you are releasing the relationship with love, thank the other person for the lessons they have helped you to learn and let them go.

8. As the balloon and its basket disappear from view, place one hand on your heart chakra and the other on your solar plexus chakra. Give yourself Reiki for at least ten minutes, or longer if you still feel a bit "wobbly" emotionally.

You may have to repeat this visualization a few times as occasionally the links are particularly strong and stubborn, but eventually you will feel as if a weight has lifted off your shoulders. You can also write down on a piece of paper "Let Reiki bring its healing and harmonizing energies to the situation of me releasing my relationship with . . . (person's name), for the greatest and highest good." Give this Reiki for five minutes each day for a week or more, or place it under a crystal that has been charged with Reiki (*see page 240*).

chapter 10

HEALING YOUR MENTAL SELF

How you feel about something and what you think about it might be quite different. To give an example, you might *think* rationally that it would be a good idea to move to a bigger house in another area because you could have a spare bedroom for guests, and since it would be closer to work and have better schools in its vicinity than your current home does. But underneath you may *feel* emotionally uncomfortable about it because you like your neighbors, the local shops are good, and you've spent the last five years getting your home just the way you want it.

YOU ARE WHAT YOU THINK

Your thoughts are energy, constantly creating your reality, and what you think about yourself is what you become; how you think life is, is what it turns out to be for you. You may remember that in Chapter 3 I talked about the energy continuum, which spreads at one end from dense physical matter to the other end which is spiritual energy or consciousness. Human consciousness is made up of a person's subconscious self, which includes their body wisdom, plus their conscious self, or ego/personality, and their Higher Self, or spiritual insight and guidance. The "self" can therefore be defined as a continuum of awareness, and every thought or emotion you have is a tiny fragment of that awareness.

As I outlined in Chapter 2, your consciousness, or thinking, feeling self, constantly creates and re-creates your cells, and because they keep replacing themselves you have the opportunity to create almost an entirely new body every year. Unfortunately, your consciousness is often locked in the past, so it keeps re-creating the same old patterns, based on the same old thoughts and beliefs about yourself, your abilities and your body. Deepak Chopra, renowned author of many books on healing, states: ". . . healing cannot be understood unless the person's beliefs, assumptions, expectations and self-image are also understood." He maintains that your thoughts and beliefs have a direct influence on the energy in all your cells—so if you change your thinking, you can change your life and even your body.

Each person's mind is filled with an internal dialogue most of the time, as thoughts, judgments and feelings ceaselessly swirl around it, and these beliefs and assumptions create your reality, your perception of the world you live in. Each person's reality is different from every other person's reality. In effect, no two people are sharing exactly the same world, because no two people share exactly the same thoughts and beliefs, since no two people have shared exactly the same life experiences.

PSYCHOLOGICAL PROGRAMMING

If you listen carefully to your inner dialogue, you will realize that much of it reflects the concepts, judgments and opinions of the people who influenced you when you were young. Just as is the case with the emotional programming referred to in the last chapter, your beliefs and ways of thinking are the product of programming that began when you were a small child. The way you think about yourself, and your beliefs about everything in your life from money, jobs and status through to love, sex and relationships, have all been founded on what your parents, teachers and other significant adults thought and believed. And just as is the case with your emotional programming, you can let go of your psychological programming, the ways of thinking that no longer serve you, and make up your own mind.

You don't have to keep thinking the same way as your parents did—indeed, it can come as quite a shock to realize that you do think in similar ways to them! We all like to believe that as adults we have formed independent judgments, based on logical assessments of the world we live in today, but as I have said before we are all products of our upbringing, so your thoughts and beliefs are likely to be either very similar to, or completely opposite to, those of your parents. You can, however, give yourself permission to change—and I use the word permission advisedly, because changing your beliefs can be quite a challenging process. You may have held them for many years, so that they have become an essential part of you, but many of the issues you may need to work on—your self-esteem, your attitude to sex, your concepts about money—will be based on ways of thinking you have picked up during your formative years, and these may be limiting you unnecessarily now.

THE POWER OF WORDS

The words you say to yourself, the words that other people say to you (especially in childhood) or that you hear on television or in films, and the words you read in newspapers, magazines and books, all have an effect on you, and on your life-force energy, or Ki. To see an example of how words can affect you, try this exercise in front of a mirror.

Stand up straight and look at yourself. Now begin to say aloud the words "I am sad," repeating the phrase at least ten, but not more than twenty times. Watch what happens to your body and listen to what happens to your voice. Your shoulders and back will begin to slump, you will probably find it a bit difficult to keep eye contact with yourself in the mirror, your breathing will become slower, you may begin to feel quite emotional, and your voice will drop and become quieter.

Now reverse the process, continuing to watch and listen to yourself, and begin to say aloud the words "I am happy," repeating them ten to twenty times. You will find that your body straightens up, your eyes become sparkly, a smile appears on your face (you may even laugh) and your voice lightens—and all because of a few words!

This demonstrates how important it is to monitor what you say. Like the words of a well-known song, you need to "accentuate the positive, eliminate the negative, and latch on to the affirmative"! I often over-hear people saying really negative things about themselves, calling themselves stupid, or saying that they can't do things, or that they'll never be able to achieve something. And of course, if you keep telling yourself such things, you'll believe them, and they will become self-fulfilling prophecies. Just try really listening to what you say for one day and you'll be astonished at how many negative statements you make, especially as you'll probably be trying to be particularly positive that day! Once you've identified the problem, however, it can be changed.

I know you've probably been brought up to be modest, but it really does pay to say nice things about yourself—if at first you feel a bit awkward saying good things about yourself to other people, then first say them aloud when you are alone. Doing this still works, and it will be good practice for being positive about yourself to others later on.

In addition, when many people talk about illnesses, they "own" them by saying "I've got multiple sclerosis," or they even take on the identity of an illness, saying, "I'm a diabetic." I'm not trying to trivialize either MS or diabetes, or indeed any other illness, but your body listens to what you say, so if you keep affirming that you have a disease, it is bound to keep on re-creating it. Rephrase such statements to something like "I've had ME, but I'm getting much better now," or "I was diagnosed with diabetes, but I'm able to control it well now." Eventually you'll be able to leave out the "label" of the disease and just say "I'm feeling great, thanks, better than ever!"

Louise L. Hay, author of *You Can Heal Your Life*, is a great exponent of positive statements about your health; she managed to heal herself of cancer using affirmations, so they can have real benefits. Being positive about your health may not bring about such dramatic improvements for you—but it might, and even if it doesn't you'll actually begin to feel better anyway because using positive language helps you to feel more optimistic.

Garden of Beliefs Visualization

This is a lovely visualization that I've adapted from one used by Gill Edwards, author of several very good books on metaphysical living, such as *Living Magically*. It will help you to get in touch with some of your beliefs, concepts and attitudes, so that you can decide whether they are still useful to you or whether they are holding you back and you need to change them.

◆ Get yourself into a comfortable position, either sitting or lying down, and start by relaxing your body by breathing deeply and evenly, knowing that with every breath you take you are feeling more and more relaxed. Stay like this for a while, then begin to use your imagination to create a garden.

◆ Use all your senses to connect yourself fully with the garden; become aware of the colors and shapes, sounds and scents around you. Notice the beautiful colors of the flowers, the sunlight filtering through the branches of the trees, the green of the grass, perhaps the sound of bird song or the rustle of leaves in the breeze, and the scent of flowers and herbs.

◆ Identify what sort of garden this is. Is it wild and unkempt, with lots of wild flowers, brambles and long grass, or is it neatly cultivated, with smooth lawns and tidy flower beds? Is there any water in the garden? Perhaps there's a fountain, or a pond or maybe a stream flowing through it where the water bubbles over pebbles and stones?

◆ Let yourself reach out and touch something: perhaps the rough bark of a tree or the velvety softness of a petal, or imagine yourself taking off your shoes so that your feet can feel the soft dampness of the grass.

◆ Use your imagination to find yourself in this garden, and begin to walk around it. This is your garden of beliefs, and everything you see or sense around you has been planted by you. Each tree and bush, each flower or herb, represents a belief or concept or attitude that you hold, and as you walk around you come across a part of the garden that holds the beliefs you have about . . . (insert here the issue you are working on—for instance, money or relationships).

◆ Notice whether the plants in this part of the garden are rich and luxuriant and well tended, or is this area choked with weeds, overgrown and uncared for? You might notice labels attached to some of the plants, and each of the labels shows you one of your beliefs about . . . (the issue you are working on). Perhaps there is a plant labeled "life is a struggle," or a thorny rose labeled "it's dangerous to love someone because you might get hurt" or even a stunted tree labeled "money doesn't grow on trees"! There may be many plants with labels, or just a few representing your major beliefs.

◆ Look now for any negative beliefs you need to release. If you need any tools to help you dig up any large plants, you will find them nearby. Allow yourself some time now to dig out any plants that represent the negative beliefs you wish to get rid of at this time. These plants have had their day, so uproot them and perhaps put them on a compost heap or burn them on a bonfire, because it is time now to make space for new, positive beliefs.

◆ When you have got rid of the plants you don't want, you will need to prepare the soil for new planting, so dig it or rake it. When the soil has been prepared, look behind you and see trays or pots of new plants. These are also labeled, but this time with new, healthy, positive beliefs, such as "whatever I truly desire is possible," or "I deserve love, and all my relationships are harmonious," or "my work is deeply fulfilling."

◆ Have fun now, planting your new beliefs. Put the biggest plants, like trees or bushes, at the back of the plot, the medium-sized plants in the center and the small plants toward the front. Enjoy the colors and scents of the flowers, the textures of the leaves, the smell of freshly turned earth, and make sure that each plant is firmly bedded in, with enough soil to cover its roots. Nearby you will find a source of water and either a watering can or a garden hose. Make sure you water all the plants properly, so that your new, positive beliefs can grow strongly.

195

◆ When you have finished, step back and inspect your work. Doesn't it look good? Aren't the plants beautiful? Congratulate yourself for letting go of old, outmoded beliefs, and feel proud of yourself for putting in all this work to replace the old beliefs with positive, optimistic thoughts and beliefs.

◆ Take a final look at this beautiful area of your garden, then begin to walk back the way you came. You may now notice other areas of the garden that could do with some attention, but you can come back another day to attend to those, so continue back to the place in the garden where you first began.

◆ Now begin to let your awareness return, sensing the chair or bed beneath you, hearing the sounds in the room and letting your eyes open whenever you are ready. Take a few minutes to reorientate yourself, then get on with the rest of your day.

REIKI TECHNIQUES FOR CHANGING YOUR THINKING

There are several specific techniques from the Japanese tradition that can help you to rid yourself of negative thinking patterns and change your thinking to a more positive and optimistic frame of mind.

Tanden Chiryo-ho

The first of these techniques, *Tanden Chiryo-ho*, is especially useful for removing poisons or toxins from the body, but that doesn't just mean physical toxins. It can also be used to rid yourself of "toxic" thoughts—that is, negative thinking and old belief patterns or habits that are no longer useful to you, and it can help to disperse depression. In Japanese, *Tanden* means "energy vessel," *Chiryo* means "treatment or remedy," and *Ho* means "treatment, method or way."

1. Sit or stand comfortably, and spend a few moments becoming centered by breathing deeply and evenly, then *intend* that the Reiki

should flow to remove any negative beliefs, pessimistic thinking or unhelpful habits from your mind.

2. Place one hand on your sacral chakra (about two to five centimeters/one to two inches below the navel), and the other on your forehead, over the brow or third eye chakra. Wait for the Reiki to begin to build up, and sense the energy in each of your hands. Hold this position for about five minutes, or until the energy balances in both hands. (Sometimes it is better to hold the hands slightly away from the body, in the aura, as this helps you to detect the energies more easily.)

3. Remove your hand from your forehead and place it on top of the other hand on your sacral chakra. Ask the Reiki to remove from your mind any negative beliefs, pessimistic thinking or unhelpful habits that are holding you back and preventing you from living life to your fullest potential. Keep both hands in place, and let Reiki flow into your sacral chakra for as long as you feel is necessary, which will probably be between ten and thirty minutes.

4. Finish by placing your hands at midchest height in the *Gassho* position and mentally give thanks for the Reiki, bowing slightly as a mark of respect.

Seiheki Chiryo

The second technique is helpful for getting rid of bad habits, or "deprogramming" negative ways of thinking. It is called *Seiheki Chiryo*. *Seiheki* in Japanese means "habit," and *Chiryo* means "medical treatment." You first need to formulate an affirmation to work on, meaning a short, precise, personal and positive statement in the present tense about whatever issue you want to work on at a particular time. Some examples are: "I am healthy, fit and vibrantly well," or "I am releasing my negative beliefs," or "I love and accept myself as I am right now." Don't worry if the statement isn't entirely true right now—the point is to project positive, optimistic thoughts, so that these can replace your existing negative thinking.

1. Sit or stand comfortably, and spend a few moments becoming centered by breathing deeply and evenly.

2. Place your nondominant hand on your forehead and your dominant hand on the back of your head, and *intend* that Reiki should flow into your thinking.

3. Repeat your affirmation over and over again for several minutes, keeping your hands in place as you do so.

4. Stop repeating your affirmation, and remove your hand from your forehead, placing it with the other behind your head. Continue to give yourself Reiki for a few minutes.

5. *Gassho*, give thanks for the Reiki and end with a bow of respect.

EMPOWERING AFFIRMATIONS AND GOALS WITH REIKI

Another way of working with affirmations is by writing them down, then holding the paper in your hands and letting Reiki flow into them for your greatest and highest good, saying the affirmations over and over again to yourself while giving them Reiki for about five minutes. If you have Second Degree you can draw all three symbols over the paper, saying their mantras in the usual order—Distant, Harmony and Power—before beginning to say the affirmations.

You can use a similar method for working on your goals and dreams with Reiki. Write down what you really want—a new job, a loving relationship, a cottage in the country, a trip to Disneyland—on a piece of paper, and be as specific as possible. Write down *all* the aspects of what you are seeking, so if you want a cottage in the country put down all the details of what you'd like it to have: the number of bedrooms and bathrooms, the type of kitchen, central heating or open fires, a small garden or acres of farmland, and so on. Then draw the Distant, Harmony and Power Symbols over the paper, saying each mantra three times.

Hold the piece of paper in your hands and *intend* that Reiki should flow into that goal for the highest and greatest good. (If you don't have Second Degree, just hold the paper and *intend* that Reiki flows into it.) Do this for at least ten minutes a day until you achieve what you want.

However, be aware that sometimes it isn't something material that you want, but the quality of life or happiness that you believe it will bring you. For instance, wanting a holiday in a specific location might be more about the rest, relaxation, fun and time with your family you think that will give you. If this is the case, then use Reiki to bring you what you *really* want, as there may be other, more permanent, ways of providing what you wish for than a two-week break in the sun.

Make sure that you *really* want something before you ask for it. Because Reiki will always work for your highest and greatest good it will help you to achieve your ideal if it is in harmony with your life path, but it may first produce results that will force you to face up to the blocks that are currently preventing you from having what you want. For instance, if you are desperate to form a loving relationship, this might be because you don't feel you're a whole person without a partner. This could indicate that you need to work on your self-esteem and ability to love yourself, so it is likely that these issues will arise before you find a partner. So you will get what you need, rather than what you want—but at least you'll be a step closer!

Nentatsu-ho

Another way of working on affirmations and goals is by using the Japanese *Nentatsu-ho* technique. Its literal translation is "method for discontinuing a concern," so it can also be used to help you to overcome illness or bad habits, and even for learning facts and figures.

1. First, decide what it is you wish to work on, then create simple, clear affirmations or goals in the present tense, as if they were already in existence—for example "I have the perfect job, which is fun, fulfilling and financially rewarding" or "I am healthy, fit and vibrantly well" or "I am releasing my need for . . . (insert any bad habit, for instance smoking)."

2. Sit or lie down, making sure you are comfortable; close your eyes and become centered by breathing slowly and deeply.

3. Place one hand on your forehead (over the third eye area) and place the other on the back of the head (at the base of the skull).

4. Call upon Reiki and ask that you achieve your goal, or be rid of the habit or illness (or whatever it is you are aiming for) for your highest and greatest good. Repeat your affirmation aloud constantly as you hold this position for several minutes.

5. Remove your hand from your forehead, but leave the other hand on the base of the skull. Spend a few minutes in meditation, still allowing Reiki to flow, and visualize yourself as fully as possible as you would be if you had achieved your goal, or "kicked" the bad habit or become healed of a particular condition. Let the image of the "new you" become as clear as possible. Turn it into a movie so that you see all the new and wonderful things that you will be able to do, have or be when you have succeeded in your aim.

6. Finally, *Gassho*, and give thanks to Reiki.

USING REIKI FOR MOTIVATION, MEMORY AND SELF-GROWTH

You can use Reiki to help your motivation, memory and self-growth without knowing the Second Degree symbols, by placing your hands in the positions suggested below for drawing the symbols over and *intending* that Reiki should flow to help you with your motivation, memory or self-growth, but the symbols do make these techniques much more effective.

1. **For self-motivation**, draw a Power Symbol over your forehead, saying its mantra three times, and *intending* that Reiki will help to increase your motivation in general, or for specific tasks.

2. **To help your memory**, either draw a Power Symbol over the top of your head or a Harmony Symbol followed by the Power Symbol on your crown and brow chakras, saying their mantras three times, and *intending* that Reiki will help you to remember whatever it is you need to remember (this can be for a better memory generally, or for specific things).

3. **To help you learn things for exams or interviews**, use the Harmony Symbol followed by the Power Symbol on your crown and third eye chakras, and also draw it over the passages or chapters or information you need to learn, silently saying its mantra three times, and *intending* that Reiki will help you to learn.

4. **For self-growth and increased understanding**, draw the Harmony Symbol, followed by the Power Symbol, on both palms, then hold your head with both hands either on your brow and the back of your head, or on both sides. Imagine the symbols entering your head and as you silently say their sacred mantras, *intend* that the Reiki will help you with your self-growth and understanding.

5. **For achieving goals, dreams and ambitions**, draw the Harmony Symbol on both hands, followed by the Power Symbol, then hold the head with one hand on your forehead and the other on the back of your head, saying the sacred mantra three times and *intending* that Reiki will help you to achieve your goals, dreams and ambitions.

chapter 11

HEALING YOUR
SPIRITUAL SELF

Your spiritual self is your whole self, of course, including your energy body, physical body, emotional body and mental body. However, healing your spiritual self is about developing your spiritual awareness, and connecting with your inner guidance. In this chapter I provide some techniques to help you in these areas, including meditation and visualization, developing psychically, working with guides and angels, and of course using Reiki.

My personal interpretation is that Reiki is unconditional love, the ultimate connection to everything in the Universe, to the Source, to All-That-Is, so I particularly like a quotation from Brian Grattan's book *Mahatma I & II—The I Am Presence*:

> What science calls energy,
> Religions call God.
> All is ENERGY.
> All is GOD.
> The Essence of God is LOVE.

DEVELOPING YOUR SPIRITUAL AWARENESS

Unfortunately, many people don't have much awareness of their spiritual self, so they spend a lot of time trying to fill an inexplicable void within themselves by seeking power, money and material success. But the answer doesn't lie outside ourselves; it is internal, not external, and it is the essence within us all—the wise, loving, powerful and creative inner core of our being, which some call the Higher Self, or the Inner Self. Moreover, connecting with it is easier than most people think, yet without this connection it is often much more difficult to find the strength, understanding and inspiration we need to carry out self-healing on the other levels of our being—physical, mental and emotional.

For some people, a spiritual "wake-up call" happens during major changes or traumas in their lives, such as a near-death experience, or the birth of a baby or the serious illness of someone close to them. At these times we become very focused, and the more superficial preoccupations of everyday life get pushed into the background, enabling us to reach a different state. For others, however, spiritual awareness grows slowly over time, usually through developing a spiritual practice such as meditation or prayer—and practicing Reiki can also act in this way.

STEPS TO HEALING THE SPIRITUAL SELF

1. Being Present
The most important element of healing the spiritual self is the ability to be present with yourself, in the "now." You cannot begin the process of healing while you are preoccupied with mulling over baggage from the past or actively scripting the future.

2. Grounding Yourself
One excellent method of becoming more present is to engage in the process of grounding your energetic system to the Earth. Here is one method of doing this:

1. Relax by sitting or lying down, and sighing deeply several times to expel any excess air from your lungs.

2. Imagine a connection forming between the base of your spine and the Earth's core.

3. Strengthen and clear this channel by drawing in Reiki through your crown chakra and allowing it to flow slowly down and then up the channel.

4. *Intend* that Reiki flows around your body, dislodging any blockages, and use the channel you have created to drain away excess or negative energy and any unwanted physical condition, sending it downward into the Earth to be transformed and recycled.

5. Imagine energy from the Earth rising up through the chakras in the soles of your feet, and up the energy meridians in your legs, into the base of your spine, and up through the Hara line to the heart chakra. This will have the effect of grounding you, connecting you to the Earth and bringing you into greater focus on your body.

6. Finally, bring more Reiki into your crown chakra, and draw it down the Hara line to your heart chakra, allowing it to mix with the Earth energy so that it forms a yin/yang symbol of balanced spiritual and earth energies.

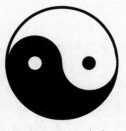

A yin/yang symbol.

7. Stay like this for several minutes while the two energies balance, bringing you into a calm, centered and grounded state.

3. Establishing a Connection with Your Spiritual Essence

After you have grounded and stabilized your body, you can bring into it more of the higher spiritual energies of your essence or soul, and this accelerates spiritual growth and awareness and promotes healing on every level. As I mentioned in Chapter 3, not all of your Soul energy can fit into your physical body—it is much too vast and infinite—but once you have been attuned to Reiki you will always be able to channel Reiki, or Soul energy, into yourself at will, raising your vibrations and becoming more and more "enlightened."

4. Connecting with Your Higher Self

There are various ways of connecting to your Higher Self. The simplest is to just find somewhere quiet where you can be alone and undisturbed for a while (somewhere in nature is especially good, like a garden, park or riverside), and then to either sit or lie down, and *intend* to connect with your inner voice. (Energy follows thought, so your *intention* sets up the connection.)

You may have some questions to ask—feel free to ask whatever you need to know. Of course, when answers pop into your mind it can initially be rather confusing, and you may just think they are your own thoughts, but one thing that can help you distinguish between guidance and your own thinking process is the speed of the answers. When you receive guidance from your Higher Self, the answer often pops into your mind even before you've finished formulating the question. Gradually you will begin to trust this intuitive sense more, and the more you trust it, the more guidance you will receive.

You can also connect to your Higher Self by using visualization like the one I've included here (*see pages 207–9*), which I've actually written for connecting to guides and angels. Some people believe that spirit guides and angelic beings are all different parts of our own Soul energy, or Higher Self, so the visualization helps you to gain insight, inspiration and guidance—whomever it is from!

Automatic Writing

Another way of getting guidance from your Higher Self is through a process called automatic writing. The method I am going to describe is one I use regularly myself, and it is really quite simple. It involves activating the creative and intuitive side of your brain—the right side—by initially writing with your left hand. (Left-handed people may be able to do it this way too, or they may initially have to use their right hand—it depends where their creative blocks are.) Having a special notebook for your automatic writing can be a good idea, as you may eventually want to refer back to guidance you received last week, last month or even several years ago. Make sure you date each entry.

1. First of all, with your pen held in the hand you usually write with, write down one or two questions you would like answered. The ones I suggest you start with are "Who am I?"; "Why am I here?" or "What is my purpose?"; and "How do I achieve that?" They are pretty profound questions, certainly, but you may be amazed at the answers you will get—sometimes people get just a few words or a sentence or two, or they may get images or symbols, but at other times they get page after page of information. Try it and see.

2. Next, hold your pen in your left hand, and write the statement "Activate right brain." This may seem pretty strange at first, but you may be surprised at how easy it can feel. If, however, what you have written is barely legible and you found it really difficult, still with the pen in your left hand write down the statement "Yes, I can." That is just giving yourself permission to access your creative, intuitive side, and it really works.

3. Then begin to concentrate on your breathing. As you breathe in silently repeat to yourself whatever question you want answered; as you breathe out continue to silently say the question to yourself. Then, in the pauses between breaths, begin to write (with the pen still held in your left hand) whatever pops into your head. At first you may get nothing, or very little or even some words that don't make any sense. Don't worry about this—it is just your ego putting up resistance and getting in the way. Accept the words and write them down without judging them—with perseverance this technique can really result in some amazing insights and guidance.

4. When you need to breathe in again, stop writing and let yourself inhale and then exhale, and during the pauses between breaths continue your automatic writing. Carry on like this until you no longer get any further response to your question.

5. You can then go on to your next question, and the process will be the same: breathe in, breathe out and write during the pauses between breaths until you are no longer getting any more information.

6. If the answers are flowing easily and quite fast, you have obviously established an easy rapport and good connection with your Higher Self, so you can stop writing with your left hand and transfer the pen into your right (if that is your usual writing hand) and carry on. You may even be able to just continue writing without waiting for the pauses between breaths, but try the full exercise several times first.

7. You can then either go on to another question, or stop and read and contemplate what you have written.

5. Connecting with Guides and Angels

Helpers from other planes can be an important part of any healing process if you are comfortable with the idea. Although all healing is self-healing, we do not exist in a vacuum and some people feel called to work with angels and spirit guides (or aspects of their Soul/Spirit/Higher Self which they choose to call guides and angels) when they do Reiki. They do this either actually when they are using the healing energy, or when they are meditating, and they may even be able to sense the presence of the helpers around them as a form of energy.

If you wish to call upon angelic beings or guides (or your Higher Self) during healing, then include them in your initial intent and invocation when you start to use the Reiki, asking your angel or guide to help you with the healing work you are about to do. Remember to thank them afterward. If you feel overwhelmed, ill or imbalanced in any way, it can be appropriate to ask for help and support, but you cannot have your lesson removed or resolved for you. What you get is perspective and guidance—the work remains yours to carry out.

You can also connect with a spirit guide or angel in a visualization, and there are many ways of doing this. You can ask and intend at the beginning of a visualization to meet a guide or guardian angel, and then imagine yourself meeting them in a forest glade or on top of a spiritual mountain, for example. If you have Second Degree, you can enhance the connection by using the Reiki symbols. Here is a very powerful connection meditation I have devised, which I hope you will enjoy trying out.

1. Make sure you are sitting or lying comfortably somewhere you will not be disturbed for at least twenty minutes. Allow your body to become centered and relaxed by breathing deeply and evenly for a few minutes.

2. Provide protection for yourself for your visual journey to the spiritual realms either by imagining yourself surrounded by a protective bubble filled with Reiki, or by imagining a Power Symbol in front of you and another Power Symbol behind you and on each side.

3. Imagine a rainbow or a ladder or staircase going up toward the spiritual realms, or draw or imagine a Distant Symbol, silently saying its mantra three times, and sending it up like a bridge or rainbow to the spiritual realms.

4. Imagine yourself walking over the bridge, and imagine Reiki flowing ahead of you, or draw or imagine a Harmony Symbol flowing across in front of you, silently saying its mantra three times to harmonize your energies with the higher vibrations of the spiritual dimension.

5. See or sense your guide or angel (or Higher Self) coming to meet you. You might see them as physical beings or as beautiful light, or just sense their loving presence.

208

6. Let your guide, angel or Higher Self lead you to a place where you can communicate with them, and ask them to provide you with helpful insights on any problems, difficulties or questions you have at this time. Give yourself plenty of time to experience this.

7. After the communication has finished they will lead you back to the start of your rainbow, staircase or Distant Symbol bridge, and may give you a sign or a gift to take back with you to the physical realms.

8. When you are about to leave thank your guide, angel or Higher Self for their loving help and inspiration. Turn and—taking any gift or sign with you—walk back down the rainbow, staircase or Distant Symbol bridge to the place where you are sitting or lying.

9. In your imagination withdraw the rainbow, staircase or Distant Symbol bridge. Go over in your mind what you saw or experienced, and examine and try to interpret the significance of the sign or gift you were given—you may find it helpful to write everything down.

10. Spend some time just doing Reiki on yourself, and meditate on the insights or inspiration you have received.

THE IMPORTANCE OF MEDITATION

Incorporating meditation into your daily routine can be a simple and effective way of enhancing your personal growth and spiritual development. Meditation is an altered state of consciousness that results in a deeply relaxed state of being, which can be used to either increase or decrease your awareness of the world around you. It allows you to experience and enjoy a feeling of being at one with yourself and the Universe, brings an acceptance of yourself and leads to a deepening of "inner knowing," as opposed to simply having acquired knowledge.

Meditation is a mental and spiritual discipline that is open to anyone who is willing to try it. Successful meditation requires practice and some self-discipline, but it doesn't have to be difficult—you don't have to sit with your legs crossed in the lotus position unless you want to, and you don't have to immediately aim for a completely empty mind! After a while you will find it fairly easy and it will become a natural part of your daily life.

In all forms of meditation there is a focus and a quietening of the mind. This aims at first simply to reduce, and eventually to eliminate, the chatter of daily life, the stresses of the environment in which we live, and so provide a haven within which we are free to connect with our inner being. It helps us to overcome the problems and illusions we create for ourselves and which we allow others to create for us, and also to overcome the habits we have formed that hold us back. Meditation allows us to go beyond the everyday, into who we really are. The art of focusing and awareness of being in the moment changes brain activity, which leads to an opening up of ourselves to the joy of the Universe. There are many methods of meditation, including:

◆ Chanting or singing using repeated simple phrases or mantras—such as chanting the Reiki Principles, or the Reiki symbols' mantras.

◆ Meditation on symbols, icons or mandalas—or the Reiki symbols.

◆ Meditation on the four elements—air, earth, fire and water.

◆ Meditation with sound such as Tibetan gongs or the sounds of nature.

◆ Meditation on the breath, counting each in-breath, or concentrating on the air flowing into and out of your nose.

◆ Guided meditation, usually called visualization, which takes you on a journey into your deeper self.

All methods of meditation are equally valid, so you may wish to try out a few in your search for the one that fits you best, or find that using a combination of meditation forms is the way for you to develop. You can start by finding somewhere quiet and comfortable where you won't be disturbed, so that you can sit or lie still for a while—and it is usually considered best not to meditate immediately after a heavy meal. It is recommended that you have your spine straight, as this aligns the chakras and enables your Ki to flow properly, but it is not necessary to sit cross-legged in the lotus position. You might like to have one or two candles lit, and burn some incense or relaxing essential oils, but these are only additions—you don't really need them.

When you are ready, just center yourself by beginning to breathe deeply and evenly, and allow your whole body to relax. Sometimes this is best achieved by tensing your muscles first and then letting them go, starting with your feet and legs, then moving to the trunk of your body, your shoulders and arms, and finally your neck, face and head.

Allow yourself to fall into a slow, regular pattern of breathing (through your nose, not your mouth). One way of maintaining focus on the breath is to count each in-breath, 1, 2, 3 and so on up to 9. After the ninth breath, return to 1, 2, 3 and count up to 9 again, continuing like this for about five minutes. When you are more used to meditating you can continue for much longer, but five minutes twice a day is a good way to start.

Once you have established a habit of meditation, you can try other methods until you find one or two you like. If you look in your local newspapers there are often groups advertising meditation classes, and there are also plenty of books, CDs and tapes available on the subject. If it isn't something you're familiar with, I thoroughly recommend that you give it a try because it is one of the best ways to achieve the calm, tranquil inner space which will help with your healing.

Guided Meditation

In guided meditation, often called visualization, you allow your Soul/Spirit/Higher Self to influence your mind and present you with new ideas and concepts, or a different way of looking at things. Often during each day something will jog us out of our limited reality and allow our minds to go somewhere else—a state we usually describe as "daydreaming," which is simply another "altered state of consciousness." Guided meditation or visualization is a much more structured, supportive and effective vehicle for achieving an altered state of consciousness, where we become open to guidance from our Higher Selves.

When you begin visualizations you may have an expectation that you should "see" things very vividly, but few people do. As an exercise, close your eyes and try to remember what your bedroom looks like. Can you "see" how the furniture is arranged? Do you "know" what color the curtains are? That's visualizing! The more often you take yourself on visual journeys, the more the focus of what you "see" will become clearer, more defined and more definite. There's no need to set up unrealistic expectations, however, so as I have said elsewhere, don't expect Technicolor Panavision Widescreen!

There are several visualizations in this book, as well as many CDs and tapes available of visualizations or guided meditations. My particular favorites are those by Gill Edwards and Sanaya Roman, detailed in the Resources section (*see page 260*), or of course you can make up your own tapes, or just let your mind lead you where it wants you to go. Choose a beautiful place to imagine to start with, such as a sunlit glade in a forest, or a sandy bay with the sound of gentle waves in the background, and then just "go with the flow" and enjoy it.

Using the Reiki Symbols and Mantras for Meditation

If you have done Second Degree, you might like to try out the following techniques.

Chanting Mantras

Sit quietly, allowing yourself to become centered by breathing deeply and evenly, with your back straight, and begin to chant one of the symbol mantras. Chanting in this way is usually done in a monotone, and if you followed the Eastern traditions you would chant the mantra 180 times. However, you can just chant until you wish to stop. When I do this I find the mantras for the Power Symbol very energizing and those for the Harmony Symbol very calming, while the Distant Symbol often inspires intuition, and the Master Symbol just feels wonderful!

Breathing Meditation with Mantras

If you are familiar with breathing meditation this will just be an adaptation. Sit quietly with your back straight, and concentrate on your breathing. As you breathe in, silently say the mantra, and as you breathe out, silently say the mantra, allowing your breathing to become deeper and slower as you do this. You can follow this practice for as long as you like, but ten to fifteen minutes is good. Of course, you can use any of the symbols, or perhaps do five minutes of breathing meditation with each.

Visualization and Breathing Meditation

This is an adaptation of the breathing meditation above. Still breathe in and out, silently saying the mantra to yourself, but in addition visualize the symbol itself. This usually induces a very profound state of meditation after about five minutes, and often produces insight or inspiration.

Stepping Into the Symbols

All of the Reiki symbols are three dimensional, having height, width and depth, so experience each of them in turn by drawing them really large in the air, imagining that they stretch into the distance, and then stepping into them. Let the essence of each symbol permeate your body and mind, and again you may experience some insight or inspiration. This is a particularly good technique to do in the open air if you can find a nice private spot.

Walking the Symbols

Imagine that one of the symbols is drawn out on the floor and step into it. Wait for a short while, until you can feel the Reiki flowing, then begin to walk the shape slowly and steadily. If you have a suitable (large) space, you might like to close your eyes, as this enhances the amount of sensation you can experience. Let yourself experience the beauty of the shape while silently saying its mantra. If you use the

Distant Symbol, you can also imagine that it is connecting you to your future self, forming a bridge through time. This can be a particularly powerful and insightful experience.

ENHANCING INTUITION AND PSYCHIC ABILITY

Everyone has some form of psychic ability, which they can choose to either develop or block. However, being attuned to Reiki can often unblock this ability, or allow you to develop it further than you would otherwise have done. This isn't anything to be nervous about, because as always Reiki works only for the highest and greatest good, so if it is the right time in your spiritual journey for you to develop your intuitive skills, you will be able to do so.

If you wish to further develop your psychic awareness and intuitive skills, work on your third eye (brow chakra) by holding your hands there and letting the Reiki flow into it, *intending* that it help you to safely and easily develop your intuition for your highest and greatest good. Alternatively, try the following exercise with the Reiki symbols. Before carrying out this exercise, first refer to the section on energetic protection (*see pages 53–54*).

1. Draw both the Power Symbol and the Harmony Symbol into each hand.

2. Hold one hand (it doesn't matter which one) on your forehead and the other behind your head at approximately the same level.

3. Alternatively, draw both symbols actually on your forehead, or in your aura, about five centimeters (two inches) away from your third eye chakra.

4. *Intend* that Reiki should flow into your third eye to awaken and enhance your intuitive ability safely and easily, for your highest and greatest good.

5. Hold your hands on your head for a few minutes, allowing the Reiki to flow.

Don't carry out this technique too often, or for too long, as it may give you headaches. If you don't feel comfortable doing it, write on a piece of paper: "I wish to develop my psychic awareness safely and easily, for my highest and greatest good." Hold the paper between your hands and give it Reiki, or draw the symbols over it, or put it in the center of a crystal grid (*see page 241*).

part four

HEALING YOUR LIFE

chapter 12

WORKING WITH THE
REIKI PRINCIPLES

In Chapter 1 I described how Dr. Usui adopted five principles for living a good life that were adapted from ancient Buddhist texts by Emperor Mutsuhito, the Meiji emperor in Japan. Normally when you attend a Reiki First Degree course you are taught the five Reiki Principles, although the versions may be different, depending upon how your Reiki Master was taught. For example, when I did Reiki First Degree in 1991 I was taught the following:

1. Just for today, do not anger;

2. Just for today, do not worry;

3. Honor your parents, teachers and elders;

4. Earn your living honestly;

5. Show gratitude to every living thing.

Another version of this was also in common use in the 1980s and 1990s:

1. Just for today I will let go of anger;

2. Just for today I will let go of worry;

3. Today I will count my many blessings;

4. Today I will do my work honestly;

5. Today I will be kind to every living creature.

These two versions were taught by two different branches of Reiki, the first by Masters who joined the Reiki Alliance, under the direction of Phyllis Lei Furumoto, Mrs. Takata's granddaughter; the second by Radiance® Technique Reiki Masters under the direction of Dr. Barbara Weber Ray, another of Mrs. Takata's twenty-two Reiki Masters. However, in the late 1990s the author and Reiki Master Frank Arjava Petter gave us access to the original version of the Principles, written in Dr. Usui's own hand, which he translated as follows:

Kyo dake wa	Just today
1. *Okoru-na*	1. Don't get angry
2. *Shinpai suna*	2. Don't worry
3. *Kansha shite*	3. Show appreciation
4. *Goo hage me*	4. Work hard (on yourself)
5. *Hito ni shinsetsu ni*	5. Be kind to others

Another translation from the Japanese is this:

For today only

Do not anger

Do not worry

Be humble

Be honest in your work

Be compassionate to yourself and others

Obviously all the versions are fairly similar, although the second of the Western versions is closer to the original. At first it is difficult to see where the third Principle, "honor your parents, teachers and elders," has come from, but it is probably just another way of interpreting "be kind (or be compassionate) to others." "Honor your parents, teachers and elders" is not just about being kind to older people! It's really about honoring and respecting everyone we meet for the part they play in our lives—parents, siblings, partners, friends, neighbors, colleagues, children, shop assistants, taxi drivers, and so on. It means acknowledging the importance of every interaction we have under any circumstances, because every person we meet is one of our teachers, whether we love them or loathe them, and every interaction is a potential learning experience, because from a soul perspective all experiences, pleasant or unpleasant, contribute to the soul's growth and development. Also, of course, if you honor (or are kind to) others and treat them well, they will honor and respect you too. What goes around, comes around!

CHANTING THE PRINCIPLES

Dr. Usui instructed his students to repeat the Principles aloud daily as a means of absorbing them into their lives, and they were seen as a vital part of his Reiki healing system. As you will have seen in Chapter 4, they are normally repeated, or chanted, as part of the *Hatsurei-ho* cleansing and meditation technique. I have given the phonetic pronunciation there (*see page 63*), so you can try chanting them in the original Japanese, which I find a really beautiful thing to do. They have a rhythm and resonance that just seems so peaceful, so they make an ideal mantra for chanting. You can repeat the same Principle, over and over again, to help you to work on a particular issue—for example, if you are finding it difficult to stop worrying about some problem, then chanting "Just today, do not worry" or *"Kyo dake wa, shinpai suna"* (pronounced kee-oh dah-kay-wah shin-pie soo-nah) might help. Alternatively, repeating all five Principles over and over again is a relaxing and meditative thing to do.

LIVING WITH THE REIKI PRINCIPLES TODAY

Although Usui asked his students to live by the Principles more than eighty years ago they are still as relevant to Reiki students, and others, today as they were then. Working more closely with the Reiki Principles can be a valuable part of your self-healing, as you gradually absorb them into your everyday life. Using meditation and the Reiki symbols will also help you to develop a deeper understanding of their meanings.

One of the methods you might like to try is to turn the Principles into positive affirmations. You can place the affirmations under your pillow, or on your lap, when you are doing a self-treatment, *intending* that the Reiki flow into the affirmations to help you to absorb them into your being. Affirmations are always couched in the present tense and in positive terms, and because some of the Principles are telling you what not to do, rather than what to do, they need to be changed a bit from the original wording. They can, for example, be as follows, although you might come up with your own versions:

Reiki Principle	Affirmation
Just today, don't anger	Today I am calm and peaceful
Just today, don't worry	Today I am carefree and joyful
Just today, show appreciation	Today I appreciate everyone and everything in my life
Just today, work hard (on yourself)	Today I am growing personally and spiritually with Reiki
Just today, be kind to others	Today I choose to be kind to everyone and everything I meet

JUST TODAY

One of the most important aspects of the Reiki Principles is the phrase "Just today," because it highlights the need to live in the moment and be aware of what is going on around you; to live in the present, in the "now." One of my favorite sayings is:

Yesterday is history;
Tomorrow is a mystery;
Today is a gift,
That's why it's called the present!

Being mindful is a Buddhist precept, meaning having your mind right here, right now, and not allowing your thoughts to wander into memories of times gone by or imaginings of times to come. Many people spend most of their time with their minds somewhere else. Their thoughts are perpetually on what happened yesterday, or last week or last year; what they wish they had said to that traffic cop, why they hadn't bought that bargain-price television when they had the chance, and so on. Or their thoughts are constantly on what might be in the future, from "what if" scenarios to what's in the freezer that they can cook for dinner tonight, or where to go on holiday, or how to get their son to swimming practice in time, and the like. While such thoughts are spinning through your mind, you are not living life as it really is; you are on autopilot.

Eckhart Tolle, in his book *The Power of Now*, states, "Wherever you are, be there totally." He proposes that for some people the "here" is never good enough, so they need to escape it with thoughts of what used to be or what might have been if things had worked out differently. He suggests that if you find your "here and now" intolerable and it makes you unhappy, you have three options: remove yourself from the situation, change it or accept it totally. A fairly stark answer, maybe, but it is about taking responsibility for your life and accepting the consequences. Choose one of those options, and choose it now, is his proposition. And then get on with living—in the present.

There are some simple things you can do to practice "being in the now." Try this on a day when you have some time to yourself. Take an alarm clock or cooking timer or something similar, and set it to go off once every hour for eight hours. Then when it rings just pause for between three and five minutes and practice being aware, using all your senses—look around you, noticing colors, shapes, light and shadow; listen to any sounds; touch things around you, noticing

223

different textures and temperatures; really breathe in the scents and smells around you. If the alarm goes off while you are eating or drinking, really allow yourself to appreciate the taste and texture of whatever is in your mouth.

This may sound like a very simple exercise, and you may question why you need to do it more than once in a day, but it can be really profound to do it every hour because you become more sensitive to the various sensations as the day progresses. It's a good thing to repeat when life isn't going too well, or when you know you've just been rushing around for days on end, because it brings things to a full stop. And it helps you to remember that you are a human being, not a human *doing!*

Choices and Changes Visualization

Here is a simple visualization that might help you with any choices you need to make. Think about a particular situation, and the various options you have (not more than three, preferably). For example, if you are unhappy in your current job, your options could be to stay in the same job, to stay with the same company but maybe try to work in a different department or to get a job somewhere else.

◆ First, get yourself relaxed in the usual way, sitting or lying down comfortably, and allowing your breathing to become deep and even, then *intend* that there is a bubble of light around you, and fill this with Reiki so that it forms a protective shield around you.

◆ Ask Reiki and your Higher Self to help you with your decision, and take yourself on an inner journey. Imagine yourself walking down a corridor, and at the end of the corridor there are two or three doors. Spend a few minutes examining the doors. What are they made of? What color are they? Do they look substantial? Decide which door represents which option. (You can have another door, if you wish, representing "something else," which can simply mean some other opportunity that may soon come up.)

◆ Open each door, one by one, and either look at what appears on the other side from the threshold, or actually step into that "reality." You may get a vision of what it would be like, or what you see may be just symbolic. For example, you might see a beautiful sunny landscape through the door representing one possible option, which would be a pretty good sign! However, you could alternatively get a stormy scene, perhaps indicating problems if you go ahead with that option, or just fog, which usually means that now is not the right time to make a particular choice. Neither of these visions necessarily means no, but it could mean that you need to wait a while.

◆ After you've had time to explore what is behind one door close it carefully and go on to the next. When you've seen what is behind each door, imagine yourself walking back along the corridor to the place where you first began, then let your awareness of your surroundings return—the chair you are sitting in or the bed you are lying on, and the sounds in the room. When your awareness has fully returned take a few deep breaths and then write down what you experienced. Sometimes you don't get instant insights into the meaning of what you've seen in a visualization, so writing about the visualization helps you to remember it if you want to check it in a day or so. Finish by giving yourself some Reiki for five or ten minutes.

DO NOT ANGER

Anger may feel like the only option under some circumstances, but it can be a very destructive emotion that often hurts us almost as much as it hurts those we direct it against, who are often the people we care about the most. Anger is usually triggered when someone or something fails to meet our expectations, or even more importantly, when we do not come up to our own expectations. However, like any other emotion, anger is actually a conscious choice, a habitual response you have developed (*see also page 176*).

225

Expressing anger toward someone rarely achieves anything other than to make you both feel bad, but you *can* break the cycle and choose a different response instead. You can find healthier and safer ways of expressing the frustration that usually lies behind the anger by turning the emotion into creativity, or going for a brisk walk or doing that very old-fashioned thing: counting to ten before you speak! Sometimes a short pause is all it takes to defuse a situation and allow you to talk calmly, in an assertive and adult way, rather than sliding into belligerence and aggressiveness.

The next time you feel angry just pause for a moment and ask yourself, "Why?" What is going on? Is this a replay of something that has happened over and over again? Are you angry about the thing you think you're angry about—such as a partner's insulting comment in front of your friends—or is there something deeper going on, like a general dissatisfaction with your relationship? It's only by asking yourself these sorts of questions that you will begin to unravel the issues that are triggering the emotion of anger, and then you can begin the healing process, so you can choose not to be angry—just for today. You can also use Reiki and visualization to help you to develop forgiveness and understanding of yourself and other people.

Forgiveness Visualization

Try this by thinking of one person to start with, although when you're more practiced at it you could visualize a small group of people, such as some members of your family, or a number of work colleagues.

◆ Settle yourself comfortably and relax by breathing deeply and evenly. In your imagination create a bubble of light around yourself, and fill it with Reiki so that it forms a protective shield around you. When you are ready, imagine yourself on one side of a fast-flowing river. Take some time to make the image as real as you can—it can be a river you know, or one you just imagine— but try to see and feel and smell the whole scene: the grass or sand or pebbles on the river bank, the blue sky and warm sun, the smell of wild flowers, the sound of the running water and bird song.

◆ When you have the picture firmly in mind, look across to the other side of the river and see or sense a person standing there. This is a person with whom you have felt angry, and with whom you have decided to connect with in this visualization. Let the picture fill out, so that you see what they are wearing, and maybe see the expression on their face.

◆ Now ask Reiki and your Higher Self to help you to develop understanding and forgiveness toward this person, and toward yourself, and see or sense a bridge beginning to form between you, over the river. It may be very wispy to begin with, but gradually a good, strong bridge is created. It may appear to be made of brick or stone, wood or metal, or it may even be constructed of stepping-stones, but now there is a connection between the two sides of the river. If it still doesn't look solid, ask Reiki and your Higher Self to help again by giving you confidence and allowing you to trust the process. (If you have Second Degree, you can imagine the Distant Symbol stretching out in front of you to create the bridge.)

◆ Next, step onto the bridge and begin to walk across it, but pause in the middle. Hopefully the person on the other side has also started to walk across it toward you, but if not just wait a little longer and imagine Reiki flowing out of your hands and filling your aura, and spreading out in front of you across the bridge to encompass and enfold the other person. Ask Reiki to heal the differences between you, to create harmony and calm. (You can use the Harmony Symbol followed by the Power Symbol for this, too.)

◆ When you can meet in the middle of the bridge, which is a neutral space for you both, allow the other person to say whatever they need to say, without judging it. You are talking soul to soul, so what the other person says is the truth as they know it, even if it is not the same as the truth as you see it. When they have finished talking, speak your truth to them and ask that Reiki flow into the situation to help you to create an atmosphere of forgiveness and trust. This may take a few minutes, but be patient and eventually you will feel a spread of calmness throughout your body, and will know that you have forgiven each other at a soul level.

◆ Imagine yourselves shaking hands or hugging each other, as appropriate, and smile and thank them for being present. Also thank Reiki and your Higher Selves for being present and helping in this situation. Then turn and walk back to your side of the river, step off the bridge, and let the bridge slowly dissolve. Wave and smile at the person on the other side of the bank, then gradually let your awareness of the present return, as you feel the chair or bed beneath you, and hear the sounds in the room. Write down what you have experienced, so that you can reach even greater insight and understanding at a later date. Finish by giving yourself some Reiki for five or ten minutes.

DO NOT WORRY

Worry is linked to fear of the future and the unknown, and is often a response to a "what if" scenario; to something that might happen, but which nine times out of ten doesn't. Being a "worrier" is another habit we can get into, yet no matter how much worrying we do, it will never achieve anything or change anything; it just makes us feel awful. Whatever problem or situation you are worried about, if there is some action you can take to improve matters then take it, but if there is nothing you can do about it then there is really no other option than to "let go and let flow."

Fear is often based on negative beliefs about life or the world, so for example if you have a general belief that life is a struggle, or that the world is a dangerous place, it will color your judgment about what happens to you and will become a focus for worrying about lack of money, losing your job, being alone or having your home burglarized. Other fears are more hidden, however. Sometimes we're afraid of things because they might be good to start with, but we have a belief that good things often turn sour; for example, we might avoid becoming involved in a relationship because even if we find our "soul mate" we believe it might still go wrong, and then we'd feel even worse.

The trouble is that we like to be in charge of our lives, but very few things are really under our direct control. Another of my favorite phrases is "If you want to give God a good laugh, tell him/her your plans!" But as long as we continue to struggle and strive to bring things under our control, we are just creating an energy cycle that makes things worse—"what you resist, persists." However, there's no point in just squashing your fears down. Instead, try to become aware of what you're really afraid of or worrying about, and then send love and Reiki to that fearful part of yourself.

You can also visualize what it is you're afraid of—such as a visit to the dentist, an interview or even something really serious, like the death of a parent, if that is something that is constantly on your mind—and in your imagination see yourself coping with it. Also, whenever you have a fearful thought, try smiling, because psychology can follow physiology—or in other words if you change your body you can change your mind. Try it. It's really hard to worry with a smile on your face! If you can just let go and stop worrying about the situation, you'll feel better, and often the solution will turn up quite unexpectedly—very few things actually turn out to be as bad as we've anticipated. So you can choose not to worry—just for today.

Discover and Talk to Your Fear(s)

You can also use Reiki and visualization to help you discover and calm your fears, and to develop hope and trust. Try this visualization.

♦ You are going on an inner journey to discover and talk to one or more of your fears or worries, so take a few moments to place yourself in a bubble of light and fill it with Reiki, *intending* that it protect you from any harm at all levels.

♦ Next, imagine yourself on a path at the edge of some woodland. The sunlight is filtering through the trees and warming you and lighting the path. On either side of the path is a carpet of bluebells, and they look and smell beautiful; you begin to walk along the path into the wood. As you continue walking, ahead of you there is something blocking your path. At first you can't quite see what it is, but as you draw closer it becomes identifiable. It may be an object like a large boulder or a tree trunk across the path, or it may be a person or an animal or bird, or a being of light, but it is not threatening in any way, and you feel quite safe, because you know you are protected by Reiki, and you know it is appearing in this visualization in order to help you.

♦ When you get quite close to whatever is blocking your path, pause for a few moments, and mentally ask the blockage what fear or worry it symbolizes. Whether it is a person, a creature or an inanimate object, it will be able to communicate with you at an energetic level, so just wait until you begin to get impressions and information. These may be words or images, sounds or symbols, but allow yourself to accept whatever is said without judgment or denial.

♦ When you are no longer getting any answers to your question, ask the blockage for guidance on what you can do to overcome this fear or worry, and listen and watch again for any answers. When you have finished receiving impressions, thank the blockage for its help, and ask it if it would like some Reiki in return. If it says yes, then imagine and *intend* that Reiki flows out of your hands to encompass the blockage in its healing, harmonizing energy, and you will notice that the blockage begins to fade and become fainter, until it finally disappears and your path is clear again.

♦ If the blockage does not wish to receive any Reiki, ask it to move aside and let you pass and it will usually do so. If it refuses to move aside, this means that you have further healing to do on the issue, but you will have received information to help you with this; thank it again, and turn back along the path to where you first began, at the edge of the bluebell wood.

♦ Let your awareness begin to return, feeling the chair or bed beneath you and the sounds in the room, and write down what you have just experienced, together with any insights that occur to you as you are writing, and any information, advice or symbols you were given by the blockage you encountered. Finish by giving yourself some Reiki for five or ten minutes.

SHOW APPRECIATION

Society today seems to have a culture of wanting bigger, better and more, and it's easy to forget just how much we already have. It is important to value and appreciate many things in our lives and to be grateful for our many blessings—to develop an "attitude of gratitude," rather than just taking things for granted. Few, if any, people reading this book will have no roof over their head at night and no food in their stomachs, so even on your worst day you still have plenty to be thankful for—and that's not meant as a pious comment; it's just a fact of life.

There is so much beauty, so much fun, so much pleasure to be had if we just take time out of every day to stand and stare—at the beauty of a flower or a glorious sunset; at the joy and laughter of a child at play; at the delicious taste and aroma of something as simple as a piece of fresh fruit. This is about developing an awareness of life and what it means to live it. Of course there will be ups and downs, happiness and sadness, but every experience is valuable because it helps to make you who you are.

So take a little time, every day, just to appreciate what you have and what is around you—for example, at the end of every day think of at least five things to be grateful for from that day, and write them in a journal. By the end of one week, you will have a list of thirty-five things to be grateful for, and by the end of a month, give or take a few repetitions, you'll have 150! And one of the good things about this is that you will naturally begin to feel happier and less concerned about what you haven't got. Also, the law of abundance says that the more gratitude you demonstrate, the more abundance the Universe will shower on you, because of course you are thinking positively and positive thought energy attracts positive things. So just for today, show appreciation and give thanks for your many blessings.

You can also use Reiki and affirmations to help you to learn to trust in the abundance of the Universe and to develop your own belief in your deservingness of love, beauty, peace and anything else you need or desire.

◆ Sit quietly and center yourself, breathing deeply and evenly, and intend to draw in Reiki through your crown chakra until it fills the whole of your body and you can feel it tingling in your hands.

◆ Place your hands on or near your base chakra (hand position 17 in the "Whole Body, Whole Self" treatment) and begin to speak any of the following affirmations out loud—or you may come up with some affirmations of your own. Repeat the same affirmation at least twenty times, *intending* that Reiki's healing energy will flow into the affirmation to bring its energetic vibrations into harmony with your own vibrations, for your highest and greatest good, that is to attract what you desire, providing it is right for you.

I deserve love and I attract loving respect from everyone I meet.
My life is filled with love, beauty and peace.
The Universe is totally abundant, and it showers me with good.
I love myself, I love my life and all is well in my world.
I now attract to myself all that I need and all that I desire, for my
   highest good.

WORK HARD

In Dr. Usui's original Principles this was intended to mean work hard on yourself, or in other words, work on your personal and spiritual development with Reiki and meditation, so giving yourself a Reiki treatment and carrying out the *Hatsurei-ho* every day would be a good place to start! Of course there are other ways to help your growth and development: reading inspirational books, learning yoga, t'ai chi or various types of meditation practice, spending time in nature, study-ing academic subjects such as psychology or theology, and so on. But the essence here is that this is a personal journey; it should be what you want it to be, and at the pace you set for yourself.

Another aspect of this, however, is to do with the wider influence of work in our lives, from paid employment to everyday tasks and how we carry them out. Do we do our work willingly and with a good heart, or are we reluctant, only doing our work because we have to, or because it is the only way we can see to earn a living? It is important to respect any work that we have chosen for ourselves and to honor ourselves by doing our best to create a feeling of satisfaction in it.

All work is valuable to the extent that we choose to value it, so it is possible to take satisfaction from even the simplest tasks, and to be willing to do everything to the best of our ability. There is an old Zen Buddhist saying: "Before enlightenment chop wood, carry water; after enlightenment, chop wood, carry water." No matter how spiritual your life may become, you will still need to work in some manner to feed yourself, clothe yourself, keep yourself warm and live comfortably.

Being honest in your work means being honest with yourself, as well as with others—it means accepting yourself for who you are. We often confuse what we *do* with who we *are*, taking our sense of identity from the kind of job we have—or do not have. What we need to remember is that we are human *beings*, not human *doings*. We are *all* valuable and special; every life, every person has a role to play in the whole and we all impact on each other in many different ways, so just for today, work hard on your personal growth and spiritual development, and honor and value yourself as the wonderful person you truly are.

So that you can *live* what you *love*, use Reiki and meditation to discover your life's purpose.

Discover Your Life's Purpose

◆ Start by sitting or lying down comfortably, and steady your breathing until it is deep and slow and you feel centered. Then begin to fill yourself with Reiki from head to toe, until you can feel the Reiki vibrations in your hands, and you can sense that it is flowing all around you, within your body and outside your body, in your aura, raising your consciousness and providing a protective bubble around your aura.

◆ Next, imagine yourself somewhere beautiful, like on a beach, or in a flower-filled meadow, or a sunlit forest glade, and spend a few moments connecting with that image with all your senses.

◆ Then imagine that a little way in front of you is a ladder, or a rainbow, or a beam of light coming down from way, way up high; walk toward it and begin to climb up the ladder, or allow yourself to slide up the rainbow or beam of light. (If you have Second Degree, you can imagine that the ladder or beam of light is the Distant Symbol, connecting you with the higher realms.)

◆ As you climb higher and higher, you become aware that your body is becoming lighter and lighter, until you realize that while you are still recognizable as you, you no longer have a dense physical body but a body of beautiful, rainbow-colored light. As you reach this realization, you also reach another higher dimension. Waiting for you are some other wise beings of light, and you can feel the happiness and unconditional love flowing from them as they welcome you.

◆ You follow the wise beings to a place where you can all sit together, and they invite you to ask whatever you need to ask. On this occasion you have come to ask about your life purpose, and how much progress you have so far made on your life path, and what else you need to do to fulfill your purpose and your potential in this particular life. Give yourself plenty of time to receive the replies, which may be in words or images, symbols or physical objects, or even charts or maps showing where you are now, and where you are going. If you are presented with anything you don't understand it is OK to ask for an explanation—these are high spiritual guides including your own Higher Self—and their intention is purely to help you as lovingly as they can.

◆ When you sense that you have been given all the information that is there for you at this time, thank the beings of light for their help, and let them lead you back to the top of the ladder or rainbow or beam of light, but know that you may return here whenever you wish to ask for guidance. With a final wave good-bye, allow yourself to slowly descend until you reach the bottom of the ladder, rainbow or beam of light, and spend a few minutes in that beautiful place you have created, remembering what you have experienced.

◆ Then allow your awareness to return to your body, feeling the chair or bed beneath you, hearing the sounds in the room, and if you feel a little woozy, just clap or shake your hands for a moment to bring you back into full awareness. Write down what you have just experienced so you can examine it a few times to gain as much insight and inspiration from it as you can. You may find that you have been given a full life plan, or just one or two points, or the first time you do this visualization you may just get a feeling of deep peace—but persevere, and in time you will get the information you are seeking about your life path and life purpose. Finish by giving yourself Reiki for five or ten minutes.

BE KIND TO OTHERS

It may seem an obvious statement, but if you are kind to other people they are usually kind to you. This seems all the more reasonable when you consider that, at an energetic level, we are all connected. As your consciousness is raised with Reiki you become more aware that every living thing is a part of you, and that you are a part of it and that everything is a part of the Divine, God, the Source or whatever you choose to call it.

The realization will come that there is no place for prejudice, judgmentalism, cruelty or indifference in a world where we are all connected, all a part of the whole, all One. All people, animals, birds, insects and plants—and even the planet itself—have a vital role to play and should therefore be valued, respected and treated with kindness. So just for today, be kind to everyone and everything—including yourself.

You can use Reiki and visualization to help you connect with all forms of living energy, and as a nurturing and loving experience for yourself. This visualization is probably best undertaken in the open air, somewhere you can connect with nature, such as a garden, a park, by a river, in a wood or on a seashore.

Connection

◆ Start as usual by finding a comfortable place to sit (or lie, because lying down on the earth can be a very grounding and connecting thing to do). Breathe deeply and evenly until you feel you are centered, then begin to fill yourself with Reiki, breathing it into your lungs, and breathing it in through your crown chakra, until you feel that the whole of your body is filled with Reiki.

◆ Then breathe in even more Reiki and spread it out still further, until it fills the whole of your aura, remembering that your aura goes in all directions—above you, below you, and on all sides—so it is connecting you with the earth below, the sky above, and all your surroundings: grass, trees, flowers, water, sand, pebbles, soil or whatever is there.

◆ As you sit or lie on the earth, ask the Reiki in your aura to flow into the Earth, and into all the plants, rocks or water near you, to bring its healing energy to the Earth and all that is natural (including any small creatures nearby), for the greatest and highest good. If you sense any resistance from anything (although this is unlikely, it can happen), gently imagine the Reiki flowing over that object, not into or through it, and mentally apologize for any intrusion. Just let the Reiki flow for as long as you wish, from five minutes to half an hour or more.

◆ When you are ready, allow yourself to sit up or stand slowly. You may find that you feel quite "spaced out"; if you do, then clap your hands or stamp your feet to bring your awareness fully back into your body, then finish by giving yourself Reiki for five or ten minutes.

chapter 13

HEALING YOUR LIFE

Throughout this book there have been lots of techniques to try out for your self-healing, but "no man (or woman) is an island," as they say, so with Reiki you have an opportunity to spread healing into your personal world to help you create physical, mental, emotional and spiritual health for yourself, because the more Reiki there is in your life, the better. For instance, if you have family or close friends around you, why not suggest that they also become attuned to Reiki? Then you can help each other by swapping Reiki treatments on a regular basis, and perhaps meditating together, which can be a nice thing to do.

If you are a Reiki Master you could also consider attuning your pet dog or cat into Reiki, having first "tuned in" to the animal to ask its permission. Animals have Soul energy too, so they can use Reiki, and you will find a new and stronger link between you and your pet— often if you're poorly or a bit down in the dumps, you'll feel the Reiki coming from your cat, curled up on your lap, or from your dog with its paws resting on your feet. It's lovely!

You can Reiki everything you eat and drink to enhance its life-force energy, plus any medications or remedies you take to aid their effectiveness and reduce any potential side effects. You can spread Reiki around your home, your garden, your car or any spaces you regularly occupy. If you have Second Degree, you can use the Power Symbol for this, but if not, then just sit or stand in the space you want to fill with Reiki, and intend that Reiki flows out of your hands to fill the space with its healing, harmonious energy. (See Chapter 4 for energy-cleansing techniques, which it would be good to do first.)

237

You can hold objects and let Reiki flow into them, too, although this works best if you have Second Degree and can use the Power Symbol. If you do, use it regularly over just about everything in your home with the *intention* of filling it with Reiki so that not only will it function even more effectively, but it will also emanate Reiki—consequently, as you walk around your home or other spaces you regularly use, you will always be soaking up Reiki.

The obvious things to use Reiki on are your bed, armchairs and sofa, dining chairs and table, desk, chair and computer if you have one, because you will spend lots of time with these things, but you can be even more creative. Try using Reiki on all your electrical equipment such as your television, CD, video or DVD player, washing machine, and of course your telephone, cell phone or pager; and on your kitchen equipment like your dishwasher, stove, microwave oven, tea kettle and toaster. You can use Reiki (with or without the Power Symbol) on personal items, such as your clothes, jewelery, toiletries and cosmetics, and using it on things like your car, motorbike, furnace or lightbulbs is said to make them more fuel efficient (well, it seems to work for me!). Don't just limit yourself to what I have suggested. Be creative!

USING REIKI IN YOUR ENVIRONMENT

I mentioned earlier that your energy field could be affected negatively by other energies such as television and radio waves, cell phone signals and so on (see Chapter 7). Unfortunately there is very little chance of getting away from such electromagnetic pollution these days, especially in built-up areas. Even in the countryside there are overhead electricity cables, television and radio transmitters and cell-phone towers to contend with, so your physical and energy bodies are being bombarded constantly with electromagnetic energy and no one really knows the long-term effects this can have. My guess is that it won't be good!

One solution is to move as far way as possible from all of the above, which is what I have done, but that clearly isn't possible for everyone. So what *can* you do to protect yourself from electromagnetic pollution? Start by limiting the effects in your own home. When not in use, don't just switch off electrical appliances or leave them in "stand-by" mode—take the plug out of the socket. This is especially important in the bedroom, where many people have televisions, music centers and even computers, which they leave on "standby" even while they are asleep, and where their radio alarm clock (battery ones are safer) and cell phone may be just inches away from their heads.

Plants and crystals help to absorb negative electromagnetic energy, so inside place quartz crystals on, or near to, electrical equipment that you spend time with, such as televisions and computers (but remember to cleanse the crystals regularly and charge them with Reiki) and have plenty of houseplants around. Outdoors, if possible, plant trees or large bushes between you and any offending masts, transmitters or electrical substations, and create a continually resonating crystal grid (*see page 243*) around your whole property, including your gardens if you have any. Also, use your thought energy to visualize a clear shield around your home—a sphere, pyramid or cube, whichever best suits the shape of the property—and fill it with Reiki, and think, believe and *intend* that the edge of the shield protects you from any damaging levels of electromagnetic energy from nearby sources.

USING REIKI WITH CRYSTALS

Using Reiki with crystals is not usually seen as a part of traditional Reiki, but many Masters and Practitioners find crystals a useful and attractive addition to their healing work. Crystals and gems have been used throughout history for their healing qualities and beauty, and each type of crystal has different energy-balancing and vibrational qualities.

Most of the popular crystals are forms of quartz, and its unique crystalline structure seems to be ideally suited to holding healing energy. The most commonly used crystals for this purpose are clear quartz, rose quartz and amethyst. When choosing crystals to buy, hold the intent or purpose of "healing" in your mind as you select them and you will intuitively be drawn to the right type of crystal for you to work with.

239

Cleansing Crystals

The first thing to do, before using any crystal, is to cleanse it properly. The easiest way to do this is to hold the crystal under cold running water, and then let it dry naturally in full sunlight, although using mineral water or holding a crystal in a swiftly flowing stream or river is considered to be better than using tap water, which contains chlorine and other chemicals. Sometimes you will be advised to place crystals in salt or salt water but this isn't really a good idea because the salt can affect some crystals. You can also use Reiki to cleanse crystals simply by holding a crystal in your hands and *intending* that the Reiki should cleanse it. If you have Second Degree, draw the Power Symbol over the crystal, say the symbol's sacred mantra three times, and say, "I cleanse this crystal with Reiki" three times.

Programming Crystals

The next stage is to "program," or charge, your crystals with Reiki. Do this by holding the cleansed crystal in your hands and *intending* that it should hold the healing energy and release it when required. If you have Second Degree, you can draw the Power Symbol over the crystal, say its sacred mantra three times and then allow Reiki to flow into it to program it.

Ways of Using Crystals

You can then use the charged crystal in several ways, such as placing it on a chakra during a self-treatment or while meditating, or carrying it around with you in a pocket or bag to aid your own healing or giving it to someone else who needs healing energy. You can also write down any problem you are experiencing on a piece of paper and place it under the crystal, *intending* that the Reiki will flow constantly into the problem to create healing for the highest possible good, but if you do this you will need to cleanse the crystal and reprogram it once a week to maintain the strength of the energy.

Creating a Crystal Grid

Another very effective way of using crystals is to create a crystal grid, which simply means grouping four, eight or twelve crystals around a central crystal. Clear quartz is the most versatile crystal, so it is probably the best crystal to use. You will therefore need to collect four, eight or twelve evenly sized pieces of quartz with "points" at one end (*see illustration below*), although you can use double-pointed wands—that is, with points at both ends—but these are more expensive. You will also need a crystal for the center of your grid—a shaped crystal can be good here, such as a pyramid, or sphere, because then the sides of the central crystal will reflect the Reiki back and forth to the outer crystals, but other shapes will do as well.

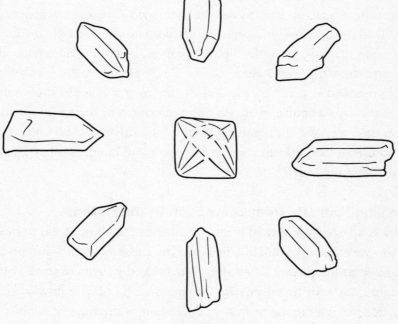

A crystal grid.

Placing the points facing the central crystal concentrates the energy into the center of the grid, while placing the points facing outward allows the energy to dissipate over a wide area. Using a crystal grid enables you to place something in the center (under the central crystal) so that it receives continuous Reiki—although you will need to cleanse the crystals and "top up" the Reiki regularly. You can therefore use a grid to empower goals or affirmations; to send distant healing to an individual (or to yourself) or to a list of people; to send healing to a single situation or multiple situations; or to send Reiki to a future or past event. Of course, always remember to add "for the greatest and highest good" whenever you are using Reiki.

To empower your crystal grid, first ensure that all the crystals have been thoroughly cleansed, then pick up each crystal individually and hold it in your hands for a minute or two, *intending* that it be filled with Reiki. If you have Second Degree, draw all three Reiki symbols over each crystal, *intending* that they be filled with an unlimited supply of Reiki, to be used for healing purposes. (Reiki Masters can also use the Usui Master Symbol.)

Finish by placing the crystals in their grid formation and either hold your hand over the central crystal, *intending* that Reiki flow into the grid, or draw the Power Symbol over the grid, saying its mantra three times and *intending* that Reiki empower the grid. After that, the grid is ready to use, but do try to put it somewhere safe, where it won't be disturbed. Placing the crystals in their grid formation on a tray and then putting it on a high shelf, or even on top of a wardrobe, would keep it away from pets and children—but please don't let it get dusty!

Healing Your Life from Conception to the Present

This is an excellent way of using a crystal grid to allow Reiki to flow into every year of your life, from the moment of your conception right up to the present. The easiest way to do this is to use small Post-it notes, and start by writing on the first one: "Let Reiki flow to create deep healing in me from my conception to the time of my birth, for my greatest and highest good." Then place the Post-it note (folded if necessary) under the central crystal and repeat out loud what you have written, holding your hands over it and intending Reiki to flow into the crystal and the piece of paper. If you have Second Degree (which will be more effective in this technique), draw out each of the three Reiki symbols (plus the Master Symbol, if you have it) over the grid, with their mantras, and leave this in place for about a week.

At the beginning of the second week, remove that Post-it note, and replace it with the next, on which you have written: "Let Reiki flow

242

to create deep healing in me for the whole of my birth process, for my greatest and highest good." (The birth process deserves a whole week—or more—to itself, as it is a particularly traumatic event.)

On the third week replace the note with the next Post-it note, which states: "Let Reiki flow to create deep healing in me for the first year of my life, from my birth until my first birthday, for my greatest and highest good." The next week's note will state: "Let Reiki flow to create deep healing in me for the second year of my life, from my first birthday to my second birthday, for my greatest and highest good," and so on. Just continue like this for each year of your life. (I managed it in exactly a year when I was fifty!) Of course, if any particular years were very traumatic, you can give them longer than a week, and do remember to cleanse the crystals and top up the Reiki with the symbols again every week.

If the prospect of spending a whole year (or more) on a project like this seems a bit daunting, try the technique by changing the Post-it note on a daily basis, so each year of life is given one day's healing. Clearly it won't be as effective, but it is a good way to begin because you will start to notice some differences quite quickly. What often happens is that as you are treating a particular year of your life, you may dream about events that happened then or memories will suddenly come back and you will know that the healing is taking place. So when you've tried it one day at a time, perhaps you'll be more willing to try a week for each year. The technique can have amazing effects, especially if you are also doing other self-healing techniques from this book, as it helps to raise issues to the surface and therefore enables you to be better able to carry out the steps to self-healing—acknowledgment, acceptance, awareness and action.

A Continuously Resonating Field of Reiki Energy

Another way of using crystals is to set up a "Continuously Resonating Field of Reiki Energy," a technique developed by Light and Adonea, two Reiki Masters in the United States. With this method, you set up a defined area of space, such as your bed, or a room, or a whole building, to hold a continuous field of energy that will benefit you or any other life-forms in it (people, animals or plants).

Take four crystals of a similar size, and cleanse them and empower them as above with the three Reiki symbols (plus the Master Symbol if you have it). However, as you program the crystals with the symbols, say that you wish to empower each one with unlimited Reiki treatments, and state the *intention* that the field of energy between the four crystals should be stimulated each time the molecules in the crystals move or vibrate—and since there is continuous action at a quantum level in all matter, that means all the time!

Then place each of the four crystals in a different corner of a room, or on the outside corners of a house or other type of building, or on the boundaries of a garden or field, and so on. Now visualize the energy lines connecting all four crystals, that is diagonally across the center, and directly between each corner, creating an energy field that continues upward, above the ground, as well as downward, beneath the ground. Then draw or visualize the Power Symbol in the center of the resonating field of energy, say its sacred mantra, and see it spread out to empower the whole of the enclosed space with unlimited Power Symbols; repeat the *intention* that the resonating field of Reiki energy which has just been created should continue its action with each molecular vibration.

The result will be that *everything* within the space between the crystals will continue to receive ongoing Reiki, so this is excellent for your bedroom, office or work space, all your living space, your garden or allotment, and so on. Have fun with it! (It is a good idea to cleanse the crystals occasionally, perhaps once every couple of months, and then repeat the above process.)

SENDING REIKI INTO THE PAST OR FUTURE

You can send Reiki into the past to allow it to heal past events or hurts, or into the future so that it is there waiting for you, to help you with something you are planning, such as an interview. You do need to have Second Degree for these techniques, as they use the Reiki symbols, particularly the Distant Symbol to cut through time and space, bringing all time into the *now* and all space into the *here*.

Obviously, when you send Reiki into the past it doesn't physically alter what happened, but it can allow healing and forgiveness to permeate that time, which will gently alter the way you feel about it.

1. Start, as always, by becoming centered, allowing your breathing to become deep and steady.

2. Write down whatever situation you want the healing to go to, and roughly the timing, such as a family bereavement when you were sixteen, or a divorce or separation when you were thirty-five. Draw or imagine the Distant Symbol over the paper, and silently say its sacred mantra three times, sensing it connecting the you of today with the you of that time.

3. Draw or imagine the Harmony Symbol over the piece of paper, and silently say its mantra three times, sensing its healing and harmonizing energies flowing to the hurt and upset, and to the root cause and any lessons you were meant to learn from the event.

4. Draw or imagine the Power Symbol and silently say its mantra three times, sensing a strong flow of Reiki moving into that time. Allow the Reiki to flow for ten to fifteen minutes, or longer if it feels appropriate.

5. Clap your hands to break the connection, and let go of that event in your thoughts. Trust Reiki to heal it for your highest and greatest good.

6. Finally, place your hands in the *Gassho* position, and give thanks to the Reiki for its help in this situation.

Sending Reiki into the future is just as simple. If you have an event or situation coming up where you feel you would like Reiki's help, such as an interview, an important meeting or a visit to the dentist, then again, write down the event or situation and the approximate date and time and proceed in the same way as above, sensing the Reiki flowing into the future to wait for you there. You can imagine it in a bubble, hovering above the building or at ceiling level, so that when you walk into the room you can imagine the bubble bursting with a gentle "pop," and the Reiki just flowing out to encompass the whole space to create a harmonious and healing atmosphere.

HEALING PAST LIVES

In an earlier chapter I mentioned that your Soul/Spirit/Higher Self is limitless and eternal, and some people believe, as I do, that we have all had many past lives, and that these lives can sometimes have an influence on our current lives—what some call karma. This past-life healing technique is one I have developed that can produce some very powerful healing, and is probably best done in meditation. It does need the Reiki symbols, so unfortunately you can only practice it if you have Second Degree.

Karmic Healing

1. Make sure you are sitting or lying comfortably where you will not be disturbed for at least twenty minutes, then allow your body to relax and center yourself by breathing deeply and evenly for a few minutes.

2. Start by asking your Higher Self and/or spirit guides and angels to help to heal any past life (or lives) that may be producing karma for you in this life. Those angels or spirit guides (or aspects of your Higher Self) who will help you with this task may appear to you in your imagination, or you may simply sense their presence.

3. Protect yourself by imagining a Power Symbol in front of you, another Power Symbol behind you and one on each side.

4. Now visualize connecting to that life on a bridge made by the Distant Symbol—just allow an image of it to stretch out in front

of you—and send the Harmony Symbol and the Power Symbol ahead of you as you imagine yourself walking over the bridge.

5. Visualize yourself standing on the threshold of that life, and, knowing that you are protected by your Higher Self, guides, angels and Reiki, ask to be shown, in a form that is easy for you to understand, any insights which might be helpful to you now, in your present life. Give yourself some time to "see" those aspects of a past life (or lives) that are affecting you now.

6. Then *intend* that Reiki produce deep healing in that life (or lives), healing any karmic wounds in yourself and in any people whom you affected in that life, for the highest and greatest good.

7. Thanking your Higher Self, guides and angels for their help, turn and walk back across the Distant Symbol bridge and step off, turning back to face the bridge.

8. Send a Power Symbol across the bridge to seal in the healing, then imagine the Distant Symbol drawing back and getting smaller, or fading until it disappears, so that it no longer connects you with that life.

9. Draw a Power Symbol again in front of you to cleanse and clear the energies.

10. Finally, put one hand up in the air (actually do this, don't just imagine it) and bring it down forcefully, as if you were carrying out a karate chop, to finally sever any further links with that life's karma. Imagine healing the cut with another Power Symbol, love and light.

11. Give yourself some Reiki for about ten minutes, and don't worry if you feel very emotional, as this is quite normal. Allow those feelings to wash over you and then let them go, releasing the emotions with gratitude for the lessons they have helped you to learn.

INTEGRATING THE WHOLE

Throughout this book I have shown you a range of self-healing methods using Reiki and other techniques, and I have broken them up into ways of healing the body, the emotions, the mind and the spirit. But we are whole beings and of course Reiki will work on our whole selves, and it will work in an integrative way as well as on the four levels of healing. However, as a final technique I'd like to introduce an integration meditation, which also uses Reiki to balance and harmonize your whole being. You can do this meditation as often as you wish, but it would be ideal after a period of working on one aspect, for instance emotional healing, enabling you to blend the healing you have achieved into the whole and to restore balance and harmony.

Integration Meditation

◆ Sit or lie down in a comfortable position, close your eyes and begin to relax. Let your breathing become deeper and slower. With each breath you become more and more relaxed, and you can feel that relaxation spreading throughout your whole body. Your feet and legs and hips feel relaxed; there is no tension left in your abdomen, chest or back; and your neck, shoulders, arms and hands also feel relaxed. Even the muscles around your mouth and eyes are stress-free.

◆ Now begin to breathe in Reiki, filling your whole body with its healing energy, until everywhere from the tips of your fingers and toes to the top of your head is filled with Reiki, and allow yourself to connect with your body consciousness. Become aware of how your physical body feels. Sense that it feels loved and appreciated and cared for, now that you are paying attention to what it needs, listening and responding to its body wisdom, working on its self-healing and filling it with Reiki. Allow yourself to acknowledge your body as being beautiful, and value it for being the vehicle through which you can experience physical life. Accept your body just the way it is, and let yourself sense its aliveness, its growing health and fitness, and feel comfortable and happy in your body.

◆ Next, turn your attention to your emotions. What are you feeling right now? Are there any little pockets of negative emotions stored away anywhere? Allow your emotional consciousness to seek them out. Acknowledge and accept them as valid and important aspects of yourself, then bathe them with Reiki. Let its healing energy release them with love, melting away any little pockets of fear and filling the space with love and harmony and balance, until your whole emotional body feels tranquil, yet filled with joy.

◆ Now let your attention turn to your mind. What thoughts are uppermost in your mind right now? Are there any negative thoughts flashing through your brain? Allow your mental consciousness to follow any negative thoughts and track them through to their source, acknowledging whatever belief is at the root of this negativity, and accepting that while this belief may have been useful to you in the past, it is now time to let it go. Let Reiki flow into the belief, healing it and releasing it with love, and allowing you the freedom to replace it with positive and constructive beliefs that will serve you better in the future. As Reiki heals, harmonizes and balances your thought processes, recognize that you have a new belief that you are a healthy, confident and loving being with the power to create the kind of life you truly want.

◆ Next, turn your attention to your spirit, that essence of yourself which fills and surrounds your physical body, and which is linked to your Higher Self, your Soul, that which knows you and loves you unconditionally. Give yourself time, letting the Reiki flow, and just be open to feeling and experiencing your spiritual essence. Allow your spiritual consciousness to fill your body, emotions and mind, integrating them into one whole being; a being of light; a being of love; a being of infinite potential. Acknowledge and accept yourself for who you truly are, and allow yourself to connect with the Universe, with all of creation, with All-That-Is. Spend a little time in this awareness of being suspended in time and space, in this blissful state of connectedness.

◆ When you are ready, let your awareness of your physical body return; sense the chair or bed beneath you, and hear the sounds in the room. Whenever you feel able to, open your eyes and stretch your arms and legs, perhaps shaking your hands backward and forward to bring your awareness fully back into your body. Then let yourself be quiet for another few minutes, perhaps giving yourself some Reiki before returning to whatever you need to do next.

LIFELONG HEALING

I have shown you that you can incorporate Reiki into every aspect of your life—that you can use Reiki for your physical, mental, emotional and spiritual healing, leading to overall well-being. Reiki is a wonderful, spiritual energy that can lead you toward a deeper, more meaningful and fulfilling life. It is a tool for holistic healing, a vehicle for learning and a catalyst for change. It contains unlimited love, joy, peace, compassion, wisdom, abundance and even more. Reiki is the divine love and light that powers the whole Universe; it is a gift of incredible power and sometimes daunting complexity, but Reiki is available to you, and to everyone, when you are ready to take that next, exciting step on your spiritual journey—because Reiki is your birthright. Reiki is your Soul energy, and the more of your Soul energy you bring into the physical, the more you become "enlightened," and the more you will be able to recognize your life path and realize your life purpose. I wish you joy on your lifelong healing journey!

chapter 14

A REIKI RETREAT

Because modern life is so often demanding, hectic and full of activity, it is important to sometimes take "time out," to retreat from everyday "busyness" to live more simply and more spiritually, even if only for a few days. I try to do at least a weekend retreat four times a year—my favorite times are the summer and winter solstices, and spring and autumn equinoxes, because these are traditionally times for reflection and renewal. If possible, I turn one of them into a longer retreat, or choose another time, perhaps around my birthday, to get away to somewhere peaceful for a week of quiet contemplation and creativity, withdrawing from the strident demands of the telephone and e-mails, the intrusive negativity of television and newspapers.

I realize that I am lucky, because I can choose how I live and no longer have the constrictions of a full-time nine-to-five job, or the demands of a young family to intrude on my chosen "alone time." However, I believe it is possible for anyone to find a few days for themselves if they really want to—although I grant it might take a lot of organizing and quite a bit of cooperation from family and friends! Bear in mind that the benefits of a few days on retreat far outweigh the difficulties of arranging to take that time out, and when you return to your "normal" life you will feel refreshed, reinvigorated and ready to take on the challenges of living in a calmer and more positive frame of mind.

PLANNING YOUR RETREAT

The first thing to decide is whether to have your retreat at home, or whether you need to go away somewhere. If you want to get right away from all the distractions of your household, then there are many places that offer facilities for retreat. Other possibilities include renting a small holiday cottage, apartment or camper off-season, or camping in your own tent.

If you haven't experienced a retreat before, being totally on your own for twenty-four hours a day might be a bit daunting, so sharing a smile or conversation with other people over breakfast and dinner might help to balance the solitude for the rest of the time. You could therefore consider using a traditional guesthouse or bed-and-breakfast, or pampering yourself in the luxury of a hotel or health spa.

Bear in mind that the location is quite important if you go away for retreat. It should be somewhere reasonably peaceful, preferably in the countryside or on the coast, where you can walk in beautiful surroundings to help you to connect with the natural world as well as with your own inner nature.

If you have a partner and/or children and/or pets to consider, you will probably need to plan your retreat quite far ahead so that you can make arrangements for them to go away somewhere, or be looked after at home while you are away. Of course, if your partner is of a similar mind, you can do a retreat together. Being alone isn't the only way! You just need to respect each other's need for quiet space, and spend some time away from each other or being silent while together. Some of my most memorable and insightful retreats have been in the company of a friend or two, walking and meditating either alone or together, and sharing meals, sometimes in silence, sometimes in companionable chat. For a retreat based in your own home, you will need to prepare by carrying out a thorough cleansing of the space (*see pages 69–76*), perhaps also setting up a small altar in the area you plan to use for meditation, and shopping for the food you will need for your meals. To do your body the greatest good, it is best to stick to just fresh fruits, vegetables, nuts (providing you don't have an allergy to them) and water for the two days, but if this sounds too stringent, just cut out meat, poultry and fish, and limit cereals, such as wheat, and dairy products to small amounts.

A HOME-BASED RETREAT

For many people the most likely time to go on a retreat would be during a weekend. On the Friday just before your retreat, either at lunchtime or after work, shop for the food you plan to eat (lots of fresh vegetables and fruits, water and fruit juices); cleanse the space if you haven't already done so; deal with any last-minute arrangements and phone calls you have to make; cook some nourishing vegetable soup for the weekend, and so on. Try to finish by 10 o'clock, then switch the sound off on your phone, have a cold shower, and do a *Hatsurei-ho* cleansing and meditation and a full Reiki treatment to lull you into a good night's sleep to prepare you for your two-day retreat.

Below I give a suggested plan for how to use the two days. You can change things around a bit to suit your personal circumstances, and you may have to finish sooner on the Sunday if you have children who need to come home and go to bed! But the plan gives you a framework to build on—and of course even one day would be better than none.

I've also suggested that you use a "retreat journal"—it can just be a cheap notebook—to jot down your thoughts and feelings, any insights that you gain during the two days, and maybe poems you feel inspired to write or drawings that represent something that's going on for you emotionally; anything, in fact, that occurs to you. Keeping a journal is a helpful way of expressing yourself, and a retreat can give you the time and the freedom to express yourself in your own way, in writing or through other creative pursuits.

253

A Weekend Plan

Saturday

Drink at least two liters (four pints) of water during the day—still mineral or filtered water is best.

8:00 a.m.   *Hatsurei-ho*, followed by a cold shower (with a hot shower afterward, if you wish). Dress in comfortable clothes, then drink a mug of hot water with a slice of lemon in it.

8:30 a.m.   Light a few candles and some incense and meditate for half an hour.

9:00 a.m.   **Breakfast** Lots of fresh fruit—make up a platter of fruit slices, which looks attractive as well as tasting good.

9:30 a.m.   A full Reiki "Whole Body, Whole Self" treatment for an hour and a half—three to five minutes in each hand position. You might play some gentle, relaxing music in the background, too.

11:00 a.m.   Herbal or fruit tea and piece of fruit.

11:30 a.m.   Light a few candles and an incense stick, and carry out some self-healing work with Reiki (any personal projects from chapters 6 to 12). Finish with some silent meditation.

12 noon   A walk or other activity, such as t'ai chi, chi kung, yoga or swimming.

1:00 p.m.   **Lunch** One or more big bowls of homemade vegetable soup, followed by one or two pieces of fruit.

2:00 p.m.   A long walk in the park or countryside or along the coast, taking some time in a peaceful place for connection with nature and quiet contemplation/meditation. Remember to take plenty of bottled water with you, and perhaps a piece of fruit as a snack. Alternatively (depending upon the weather), spend the whole or part of the afternoon in creative pursuits such as drawing, painting, collage, writing, carving, embroidery or tapestry work.

5:00 p.m.   Herbal or fruit tea and a piece of fruit.

5:30 p.m.   Light a few candles and some incense, and carry out some meditation and/or visualization for approximately half an hour. Spend the rest of the time connecting with your Higher Self (see Chapter 11), or working with Reiki in various ways on self-healing projects—for example, with crystals.

7:00 p.m.   **Evening meal** Large salad with lots of different salad vegetables, chopped pieces of fruit, olives and nuts, with a light dressing such as olive oil and balsamic vinegar and then a big bowl of fruit salad.

8:00 p.m.   Relaxation: reading a spiritual/self-help book, listening to calming music. (No television, radio or newspapers!)

10:00 p.m.   Writing in your "retreat journal": notes about your day, about how you've been feeling, and any insights or inspirations you've had—or anything else that seems relevant.

10:30 p.m.   Cold shower, *Hatsurei-ho* and Reiki self-treatment.

Sunday

The same basic outline as for Saturday, but at lunchtime have a huge mixed salad with hummus, followed by fresh fruits, and in the evening have plenty of hot vegetable soup and a small green salad, followed by a big fruit salad.

GOING AWAY FOR A RETREAT

If you choose to go away somewhere for a retreat, you can still follow the basic outline above, but you may have to adapt it to suit the

255

timetable of the place you are visiting. For example, if you choose a Buddhist or Christian retreat center there may be set times for meditations or prayers, and for meals, which you might choose to take part in. If you are staying in a guesthouse or hotel the mealtimes will also probably have to vary, or there may be restrictions on what you can do in your room (for example, carving wood or painting in oils might prove to be a bit too messy, unless you take the right protective and/or cleanup equipment with you).

The important thing is to remember the essence of retreat, which is to give yourself time in quietness and solitude; time to ponder; time to wonder, time just to *be*, without having to rush about doing everyday tasks, or being concerned with other people's needs. Time just for *you*.

LIVING "AS A RETREAT"

If you adopt all of the Reiki Principles, especially the idea of mindfulness—"Just for Today"—then you can eventually turn your life largely into a form of retreat. Sometimes life can be too exciting and interesting to want to retreat—and that's fine. Life should be fun! But at other times you can have what I call a "working retreat," during which you adapt your working life to give it a calmer, meditative structure, such as the one I often adopt (*see below*).

As I have already said, I know I'm lucky to be able to arrange my days in the way I want most of the time, but when I'm writing a book I may not work in a traditional "nine-to-five" way (I will admit to not being a morning person!). I do put in a seven- or eight-hour day, and when I teach a seminar, that can go up to twelve to thirteen hours a day, yet I still manage to fit in all the elements of the working retreat below, usually by getting up earlier. You may need to adjust the timings to suit your own lifestyle (it may take you longer than half an hour to get to work, for instance), but if you use the following example as a framework, you can probably come up with a similar approach.

You may notice that the plan doesn't make allowances for coping with children, pets or even your partner! But with a little adjustment here and there, and perhaps putting one idea at a time into your normal working day, you will introduce a gentle change of pace into your life. Strangely, spending time on meditation, self-healing or quiet, reflective activities seems to give you more time for other things, rather than less, because you can approach the rest of your life in a calmer way. Stress can be very time-consuming.

A Working Retreat

6:30 a.m.   Reiki self-treatment.

7:15 a.m.   Quick cold shower, followed by hot shower, dressing and breakfast.

8:00 a.m.   *Hatsurei-ho*, then twenty minutes further meditation.

8:30 a.m.   Leave for work, or if you work from home then use this time for practical tasks, such as housework, washing, paying bills, and so on.

8:55 a.m.   Five-minute meditation while treating your heart chakra with Reiki. (If you can't do this in your working environment, then you could do it while sitting in your parked car, or even while you're in the restroom at work!)

9:00 a.m.   Begin your morning's work.

11:00 a.m.   Coffee break—try to sit quietly for at least a couple of minutes, giving yourself Reiki; you can do this quite discreetly, by placing your hands on your thighs, for example. Also try to substitute herb or fruit tea for coffee for at least a few days each week.

1:00 p.m.   Lunch followed by some activity, preferably in a natural green space—you could take a short walk or do t'ai chi in the park.

2:00 p.m.   Begin your afternoon's work.

3:30 p.m.   Tea break—again, try to sit quietly for a few minutes, centering yourself with some Reiki before starting work again.

5:00 p.m.   At the end of your working day, before leaving your workplace, try to find some quiet space and carry out the *Kenyoku-ho* and/or the Reiki shower to get rid of at least some of the negativity you may have picked up during the day.

5:05 p.m.   Leave for home.

5:30 p.m.   Quick cold shower to rid yourself of the rest of the negativity you may have picked up at work or on the journey home, and change into comfortable clothes for the evening.

5:45 p.m.   Period of relaxation for chatting, reading and generally winding down after work.

6:30 p.m.   Food preparation, and enjoying your evening meal.

8:00 p.m.   Relaxation—for instance reading, painting, meeting friends, theater, cinema, television or listening to music.

10:00 p.m.   Quick cold shower (especially if you didn't manage one after work) followed by a relaxing warm bath, and then *Hatsurei-ho*, Reiki projects, such as sending distant healing, some self-healing work and meditation.

11:00 p.m.   Sleep!

A FINAL WORD

It might seem like a luxury to take the time out of your normal life for retreat, but when you are on a spiritual path—and being attuned to Reiki means that you have already taken a major step on that path—it becomes one of life's essentials. If you really feel that you cannot find time to retreat, remember that finding time is a choice. For example, if there was an emergency you would find the time to respond to it, because you would reprioritize everything else in your life.

Well, needing time to yourself might not be considered an emergency, but the reprioritizing is still necessary because the *real* you needs to emerge from beneath all the trappings and dross of modern life so that you can become the person you really are inside—as I keep saying: *a human being, not a human doing!* Time to yourself in peace and silence is as essential and nourishing to the inner you as food and drink are to your physical body. Responding to your spiritual needs will enhance your life immeasurably, and make your everyday life calmer and more fulfilling. Try it and see.

RESOURCES

CONTACT ADDRESSES
PENELOPE QUEST
For information about Reiki training, courses and CDs with Reiki Master Penelope Quest, and details of her books, retreats and workshops on personal and spiritual development, please see her website.
Website: http://www.reiki-quest.co.uk
E-mail: info@reiki-quest.co.uk

REIKI TEACHERS AND PRACTITIONERS IN THE UK
For details of other Reiki Masters and Practitioners, and useful information about Reiki and other forms of healing, you can try the following organizations and websites. (These were all correct when going to press, but please check the websites for up-to-date information.)

The UK Reiki Federation
Website: http://www.reikifed.co.uk
E-mail: enquiry@reikifed.co.uk
Address: UK Reiki Federation, PO Box 71, Andover, SP11 9WQ

The Reiki Association
Website: http://www.reikiassociation.org.uk
E-mail: co-ordinator@reikiassociation.org.uk

The Reiki Council (formerly the Reiki Regulatory Working Group)
Website: http://reikiregulation.org.uk
E-mail: info@reikiregulation.org.uk

The Reiki Alliance—UK and Ireland
Website: http://www.reikialliance.org.uk
E-mail: mail@reikialliance.org.uk

The General Regulatory Council for Complementary Therapies
Website: http://www.grcct.org
E-mail: admin@grcct.org

Complementary Therapists Association
Website: www.complementary.assoc.org.uk
E-mail: info@complementary.asso.org.uk

Federation of Holistic Therapists (FHT)
Website: http://www.fht.org.uk
E-mail: info@fht.org.uk

British Complementary Medicine Association (BCMA)
Website: http://www.bcma.co.uk
E-mail: chair@bcma.co.uk

Reiki Healers and Teachers Society (RHATS)
Website: http://reikihealersandteachers.net
E-mail: info@reikihealersandteachers.net

Institute for Complementary Medicine (ICM)
Website: http://www.i-c-m.org.uk
E-mail: info@i-c-m.org.uk

National Federation of Spiritual Healers (The Healing Trust)
Website: http://thehealingtrust.org.uk

U.S. AND CANADA CONTACTS

The Reiki Alliance—Worldwide
P.O. Box 41, Cataldo, ID 83810–1041
Website: http://www.reikialliance.com
E-mail: info@reikialliance.com

Usui Shiki Ryoho (The Office of the Grand Master—Phyllis Furumoto and Paul Mitchell)
Website: http://www.usuireiki-ogm.com

The International Center for Reiki Training (William Lee Rand),
21421 Hilltop St., #28, Southfield, MI 48034–1023
Website: http://www.reiki.org
E-mail: center@reiki.org

International Association of Reiki Professionals (IARP)
P.O. Box 481, Winchester, MA 01890
Website: http://www.iarp.org
E-mail: info@iarp.org

Southwestern Usui Reiki Ryoho Association
P.O. Box 5162, Lake Montezuma, Arizona 86342–5162;
Website: http://www.reiho.org
E-mail: adonea@msn.com

The Radiance Technique International Association Inc (TRTIA)
P.O. Box 40570, St. Petersburg, FL 33743–0570
Website: http://www.trtia.org
E-mail: TRTIA@aol.com

Canadian Reiki Association
P.O. Box 54570, 7155 Kingsway, Burnaby, BC, V5E 4J6
Website: http://www.reiki.ca
E-mail: reiki@reiki.ca

Usui-Do (Traditional Japanese Reiki)
The Usui-Do Foundation, Toronto, Ontario, Canada;
Website: http://www.usui-do.org
E-mail: askme@usui-do.org

WORLDWIDE CONTACTS

Reiki Dharma (Frank Arjava Petter)
[Translations available in English, Spanish and German]
Website: http://www.reikidharma.com
E-mail: Arjava@ReikiDharma.com

Australian Reiki Connection
Website:
http://www.australianreikiconnection.com.au

Reiki Australia
Website: http://www.reikiaustralia.com.au

International House of Reiki (Frans and Bronwen Stiene)
Website: http://www.reiki.net.au
E-mail: info@reiki.net.au

Shibumi International Reiki Association
Website: http://www.shibumireiki.org

Reiki New Zealand Inc.
Website: http://www.reiki.org.nzemail
E-mail: info@reiki.org.nz

The Wellness Directory
Website: http://www.wellnessdirectory.co.nz

The Reiki Association of Southern Africa
Website: http://www.reikiassociation.co.za

Reiki Masters Association of South Africa
Website: http://www.reikihealing.co.za

World Reiki Association
Website: http://www.worldreikiassociation.org

International Holistic Therapies Directories,
Website:
http://www.internationalholistictherapiesdirectories.com

VISUALIZATION AND GUIDED MEDITATION TAPES/CDS

Penelope Quest
Websites: http://www.reiki-quest.co.uk
http://www.penelopequest.com
E-mail: info@reiki-quest.co.uk

Gill Edwards
Website: http://www.livingmagically.co.uk
E-mail: livmagic@aol.com

Sanaya Roman/Duane Packer
Website: http://www.orindaben.com

William Bloom
Website: http://www.williambloom.com

FURTHER READING

The following books are my recommendations from the many available on each subject. I have placed them under headings to make it easier to find the topics you want to pursue, but many of them cover several categories.

Reiki

Ellis, Richard, *Reiki and the Seven Chakras*, Vermilion, 2002.

Hall, Mari, *Reiki for Common Ailments*, Piatkus, 1999.

Lubeck, Walter, and Frank Arjava Petter, *Reiki Best Practices*, Lotus Press, 2003.

Lubeck, Walter, Frank Arjava Petter, and William Lee Rand, *The Spirit of Reiki*, Pilgrims Publishing, 2004.

Petter, Frank Arjava, *The Original Reiki Handbook of Dr Mikao Usui*, Lotus Press, 1999.

Quest, Penelope, *The Basics of Reiki*, Piatkus, 2007.

———, *Living the Reiki Way*, Piatkus, 2010.

———, *Reiki for Life*, Tarcher, 2010.

———, *Reiki for Life*, Piatkus, 2012.

Quest, Penelope, and Kathy Roberts, *The Reiki Manual*, Piatkus, 2010.

———, *The Reiki Manual*, Tarcher, 2011.

Reiki Council, *The Reiki Council Resource Handbook*, Douglas Barry Publications, 2010 (available through the Reiki Council).

Steine, Bronwen and Frans, *The Japanese Art of Reiki*, O Books, 2005.

———, *The Reiki Sourcebook*, O Books, 2003.

Energy, Auras, and Chakras

Braden, Gregg, *The Divine Matrix*, Hay House, 2007.

Brennan, Barbara Ann, *Hands of Light: Guide to Healing Through the Human Energy Field*, Bantam Books Ltd, 1990.

Chopra, Deepak, *Quantum Healing,* Bantam Books, 1990.

Eden, Donna, *Energy Medicine: Balancing Your Body's Energy for Optimal Health, Joy and Vitality*, Piatkus, 2008.

Edwards, Gill, *Conscious Medicine*, Piatkus, 2010.

Emoto, Masaru, *The Hidden Messages in Water*, Pocket Books, 2005.

Hunt, Valerie V., *Infinite Mind—Science of the Human Vibrations of Consciousness*, Malibu Publishing Co., 1996.

Judith, Anodea, *Wheels of Life*, Llewellyn Publications, 1987.

Kingston, Karen, *Clear Your Clutter with Feng Shui*, Piatkus, 2008.

Lipton, Bruce, *The Biology of Belief*, Hay House, 2011.

McTaggart, Lynne, *The Field: The Quest for the Secret Force of the Universe*, Element, 2003.

Simpson, Liz, *The Book of Chakra Healing*, Gaia Books Ltd, 2005.

General Healing and Self Help

Chopra, Deepak, *Perfect Health*, Bantam Books, 2001.

———, *Reinventing the Body, Resurrecting the Soul: How to Create a New Self*, Rider, 2010.

Dyer, Dr. Wayne W, *Manifest Your Destiny*, Thorsons, 1998.

Edwards, Gill, *Life Is a Gift*, Piatkus, 2007.

———, *Living Magically*, Piatkus, 2006.

———, *Stepping into the Magic*, Piatkus, 2006.

Gawain, Shakti, *Living in the Light*, New World Library, 1998.

Holden, Robert, *Shift Happens*, Hay House, 2010.

Jeffers, Susan, *End the Struggle and Dance with Life*, Hodder Mobius, 2005.

———, *Feel the Fear and Do It Anyway*, Vermilion, 2007.

Lloyd, Alexander, and Ben Johnson, *The Healing Code*, Hodder & Stoughton, 2011.

Mohr, Barbel, *The 21 Golden Rules for Cosmic Ordering*, Hay House, 2011.

Myss, Caroline, Ph.D., *Why People Don't Heal and How They Can*, Bantam Books, 1998.

Scovel-Shinn, Florence, *The Game of Life and How to Play It*, Vermilion, 2005.

Metaphysical Causes of Disease

Dethlefsen, Thorwald, and Rudiger Dahlke, *The Healing Power of Illness*, Vega Books, 2004.

Hay, Louise L., *Heal Your Body*, Hay House, 2004.

———, *You Can Heal Your Life*, Hay House, 2004.

Linn, Denise, *Unlock the Secret Messages of Your Body*, Hay House, 2010.

Shapiro, Debbie, *Healing Mind, Healing Body: Explaining How the Mind and Body Work Together*, Collins and Brown, 2007.

———, *Your Body Speaks Your Mind*, Piatkus, 2007.

Physical Body

Atkinson, Dr Mark, *The Mind Body Bible*, Piatkus, 2007.

Bloom, William, *The Endorphin Effect*, Piatkus, 2001.

Hamilton, Amanda, and Sandy Newbigging, *Life Detox*, Piatkus, 2007.

Holford, Patrick, *New Optimum Nutrition Bible*, Piatkus, 2004.

———, *The 10 Secrets of 100% Healthy People*, Piatkus, 2010.

Holford, Patrick, and Jerome Burne, *Food Is Better Medicine Than Drugs*, Piatkus, 2007.

Northrup, Dr. Christiane, *Women's Bodies, Women's Wisdom*, Piatkus, 2009.

Vorderman, Carol, *Detox for Life*, Virgin Books, 2001.

Waugh, Anne, and Alison Grant, *Ross and Wilson Anatomy and Physiology in Health and Illness*, Churchill Livingstone, 2006.

Emotional Body

Goleman, Daniel, *Emotional Intelligence*, Bloomsbury, 1996.

Hamilton, David R., *Why Kindness Is Good for You*, Hay House, 2011.

Hicks, Esther and Jerry, *The Astonishing Power of Emotions*, Hay House, 2008.

———, *Getting into the Vortex*, Hay House, 2010.

Lynch, Paul and Valerie, *Emotional Healing in Minutes*, Thorsons, 2001.

McKenna, Paul, *I Can Make You Happy*, Bantam Press, 2011.

Neill, Michael, *Feel Happy Now*, Hay House, 2007.

Pert, Candace B., *Molecules of Emotion*, Pocket Books, 1999.

Mental Body

Carnegie, Dale, *How to Stop Worrying and Start Living*, Pocket Books, 2004.

Dilts, Robert, Tim Hallbom, and Suzi Smith, *Beliefs: Pathways to Health & Well-Being*, Metamorphous Press, 1990.

Dyer, Wayne W., *Change Your Thoughts, Change Your Life*, Hay House, 2007.

———, *You'll See It When You Believe It*, Arrow, 1990.

Hamilton, David R., *The Contagious Power of Thinking*, Hay House, 2011.

———, *How Your Mind Can Heal Your Body*, Hay House, 2008.

———, *It's the Thought That Counts*, Hay House, 2005.

Leahy, Dr. Robert I., *The Worry Cure*, Piatkus, 2006.

McWilliams, John-Roger and Peter, *You Can't Afford the Luxury of a Negative Thought*, Thorsons, 2001.

Spiritual Body

Armstrong, Karen, *Twelve Steps to a Compassionate Life*, The Bodley Head, 2011.

Hicks, Esther and Jerry, *Ask and It Is Given*, Hay House, 2005.

———, *Getting into the Vortex*, Hay House, 2010.

Linn, Denise, *Altars*, Rider, 1999.

Myss, Caroline, Ph.D., *Anatomy of the Spirit*, Bantam Books, 1997.

———, *Sacred Contracts*, Bantam Books, 2002.

Roman, Sanaya, *Soul Love*, H. J. Kramer 1997.

Ruiz, Don Miguel, *The Four Agreements*, Amber-Allen Publishing, Inc., 1997.

Tolle, Eckhart, *A New Earth: Awakening to Your Life's Purpose*, Penguin Books, 2006.

———, *The Power of Now: A Guide to Spiritual Enlightenment*, Hodder Mobius, 2001.

Walsch, Neale Donald, *Communion with God*, Hodder & Stoughton, 2000.

———, *Conversations with God*, Books 1, 2, and 3, Hodder & Stoughton, 1996, 1997, 1998.

———, *Friendship with God*, Hodder & Stoughton, 1999.

INDEX

Note: page numbers in **bold** refer to illustrations.